T0186041

Disaster Victim Identification

Disaster Victim Identification: A Manager's Guide to Policy and Procedure's guiding thesis explains why disaster victim identification (DVI) must be fundamentally integrated—at the outset—into general disaster planning and operations procedures. By doing so, it allows for pre-event assessment of any risks and vulnerabilities, in coordination with planning and response agencies, so that the on-site response isn't the first time they have communicated and worked together.

The book outlines the importance of exercising, interagency memoranda of understanding (MOU), and coordination in advance to provide the best, most effective response that optimally serves both the victims and the community. DVI requires a multi-disciplinary approach and, as such, plans should take into consideration and account for possible integration of outside assistance into the general work plan and flow. By doing this, practical action and measures—sometimes coordinated impromptu depending on the nature and scale of a disaster—can be undertaken both quickly and seamlessly.

Coverage outlines the overall DVI process, its various methodologies, and how it serves as an integral part of overall disaster response. *Disaster Victim Identification* brings together the expertise of two professionals with longstanding, extensive first-hand experience in the field. This includes working at, as well as supervising coordination of, DVI response to such scenes. The book will be a welcome addition for professionals by examining what works, what doesn't, and how to maintain best practices while avoiding common mistakes.

Jay H. Levinson is a researcher at the Hebrew University and Prof. Adj. at John Jay College of the City University of New York. Since the 1990s, he has been a correspondent for the (UK) Jewish Tribune. He earned B.A., M.A., and Ph.D. degrees in Near Eastern Studies from New York University. He also studied foreign languages at Yale, Princeton, and the University of Pennsylvania. During 1972–1981, he worked for the U.S. Central Intelligence Agency, primarily on anti-terrorism targets. From 1981 to 2002, he served in the Forensic Science Division of the Israel Police (1985–1999 in Disaster Victim Identification). From 1994 to 1999, he was Chairman, Interpol Disaster

Victim Identification Standing Committee. He has lectured in more than 25 countries and has written six books as well as dozens of journal articles concerning DVI. His research interests primarily relate to media coverage of disasters, DVI management and infrastructure, and related psychological and religious issues.

Abraham ("Avi") J. Domb is Professor for Forensic Sciences at the Faculty of Law and Medicinal Chemistry and Biopolymers at the School of Pharmacy-Faculty of Medicine of the Hebrew University. He earned B.Sc. degrees in Chemistry, Pharmaceutics, and Law; Diplomas in Business management and Textile Science, and a Ph.D. degree from the Hebrew University. He did his postdoctoral training at Syntex Research, MIT, and Harvard University. Since 1991, he has been at the Hebrew University. During 2007–2012, he headed the Division of Forensic Science at the Israel Police. During 2014–2016, he served as President of the Azrieli College of Engineering. Since 2021, Prof. Domb has been the Chief Scientist of the Ministry of Innovation, Science & Technology. His research interests include forensic science, medicinal and polymer chemistry, pharmaceutical development, and drug delivery systems.

Disaster Victim
Identification

A Manager's Guide to Policy
and Procedure

Jay H. Levinson and Abraham J. Domb

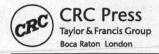

CRC Press
Taylor & Francis Group
Boca Raton London

CRC Press is an imprint of the
Taylor & Francis Group, an **informa** business

Designed cover image: © shutterstock

First edition published 2023
by CRC Press
6000 Broken Sound Parkway NW, Suite 300, Boca Raton, FL 33487–2742

and by CRC Press
4 Park Square, Milton Park, Abingdon, Oxon, OX14 4RN

CRC Press is an imprint of Taylor & Francis Group, LLC

© 2023 Jay H. Levinson and Abraham J. Domb

ISBN: 978-1-032-38500-6 (hbk)
ISBN: 978-1-032-38503-7 (pbk)
ISBN: 978-1-003-34536-7 (ebk)

DOI: 10.4324/9781003345367

Typeset in Minion
by Apex CoVantage, LLC

Contents

Figures

Introduction

In modern Western society, it is axiomatic that the bodies of deceased persons be identified. This is a common rule, essentially the product of developments in the 20th century (Daniel).

In cases of single non-criminal deaths, identification often rests with a hospital or medical authority as part of standard procedures in issuing a death certificate. There are usually few problems in routine cases, and even in instances of violent deaths, such as traffic accidents, criminal acts, or house fires, there is close contact with surviving next-of-kin or extended family in collecting ante mortem data when necessary. Given the cooperative working relationship, it is likely that a survivor's or bereaved family's concerns are addressed. There is also no over-riding pressure to deal with large numbers of other deceased persons. Hence, the family is involved in the process and can achieve closure. There is a triangle of identification interests: (a) legal standards, (b) professional methods, and (c) religious law and custom. Usually, the triangle is complete, and all interests are addressed.

Closure, the psychological acceptance of events, can only be attained when all of the family's concerns are allayed. This means that family members are fully satisfied that the identification of the deceased is not only unequivocal but also that it meets all of their needs including religious and cultural dictates. There are also other parts of concern—typically, that the standards of final internment or cremation meet family needs.

A key factor relating to the police and forensic medical staff in the identification and handling of deceased victims is "service to the public"—the need to meet public demands and requirements. This is particularly practical in the one-on-one relationship of a single death.

Disaster Victim Identification (DVI), however, is different. A generally accepted definition of disaster is an event that exceeds routine government response. The United Nations uses a different definition, stating that a disaster is a serious disruption of the functioning of a community or society, which involves widespread human, material, economic, or environmental impacts that exceed the ability of the affected community or society to cope using its own resources. According to both definitions not only is special deployment necessary. There is also a redistribution of responsibilities and job functions.

The issue of DVI arises in incidents such as disasters of numerous types, criminal acts, mass graves, terrorism, and in the context of acts of war and aggression. This book concentrates on the role of civilian management at various levels in identifying the dead, particularly in Western culture. As will be seen, there are many "partners" in the DVI process, but this book concentrates specifically but not exclusively on police functions.

This book is based on practical experience, not just theory. The first author was involved in the response to seven air crashes, countless terrorist bombings, and construction collapse. The second author served as the head of a forensic laboratory, overseeing DVI operations that involved field evidence technicians and numerous Headquarters laboratories involved in the DVI process. Their combined and complimentary experience is broad and not based on just one single incident. This book focuses on police involvement in DVI during a disaster. Many incidents in this book are not described in full detail for considerations of privacy.

General

I

Overview of Disasters 1

Disasters can be of many types (Black). Some are the result of natural causes (earthquake, landslide, storm, and flooding). Others are the result of unintentional human error (airplane pilot error or miscalculation, poor architectural design, and mistaken use of building materials). And, there are unfortunate intentional disasters (bombing, terrorism, and mass shootings). A unique category is chemical leaks (e.g., Bhopal and Chernobyl) that pose direct health concerns to responders as well as DVI personnel. Even disasters of the same cause often play out differently. In a certain sense, every disaster is unique.

As noted, there are numerous definitions to "disaster" (Al-Madhari). This book concentrates on sudden incidents. In contrast and not included here, drought and famine can cause numerous fatalities; however, generally they are without problems of victim identification.

Emergency response to a typical road accident, for example, is most often within regular working parameters, even when considering Disaster Victim Identification (DVI). A commercial air crash often exceeds routine capabilities and requires special deployment procedures. Contrary to public parlance, in professional response terms, disasters are dictated neither by an absolute number of fatalities nor by the monetary assessment of damage, although these factors do contribute to special deployment. In one jurisdiction, for example a small town or village, an incident may be a disaster, whereas in a large city, the same incident might fall under routine protocols.

DVI is a dynamic process that has changed over the years (Daniel) (Williams *et al.*). At one time, personal recognition with all of its errors (see later) was the primary method of identification, supported equally unreliably by relying on property and clothing (a distinct problem when dealing with fallen soldiers in uniform or children attending schools requiring mandatory uniforms). Slowly as time passed, methods such as fingerprints, X-rays, and odontology were adopted. Then came other new methods in the modern era, first forensic anthropology, computerized techniques, and recently most prominently DNA.

Communities in many countries are equipped to various degrees to deal with DVI, while others count on response from national authorities or even private companies. There are also countries that are essentially unprepared

DOI: 10.4324/9781003345367-2

and need international assistance. This book deals with each of these different situations.

DVI is not a stand-alone procedure. It must be integrated into the overall disaster preparedness program. It is often seen only in the response stage in which its role is obvious. DVI, however, must start much earlier, in fact from the very beginning of general disaster planning. It must initially be based on the assessment of risks and vulnerabilities in co-ordination with the community estimations, accompanied by a realistic understanding of what a disaster encompasses. Reality is that not all disaster victims will necessarily survive. That must be part of planning. Thus, DVI should be planned, taking into consideration a possible disaster scope. Although we are neither prophets nor fortune tellers, disaster scenarios including DVI must also be prepared for the unforeseen. In other words, plans should take into consideration unforeseen possible integration of outside assistance into the general work plan. Only at that planning stage can practical measures be undertaken.

Planning a Response

2

There are numerous stages when initiating a DVI program. The first step is related to general disaster management. Just as with all other planning, DVI must be part of an overall response and management protocol. The most common is the Incident Command System (ICS), the origin of which date back to 1968 and fires in Southern California. This system provides a general outline and command structure, seen as a popular albeit sometimes partial system (Buck).

Community steps, be it a large municipality or small jurisdiction, are standard—survey potential dangers, estimate their potential effect and probability, and design response, taking into consideration that the unplanned may also occur.

This stage of preparation also applies to both large and small businesses as well as governments. Even a small neighborhood grocery store should plan for fire detection, evacuation of customers through more than one exit, and communication equipment in more than one location to call for help (aided today by mobile phones that are often carried in pockets).

The crash of Pan Am 103 on 21 December 1988 in Lockerbie is a blatant example of a totally unforeseen event for which there was no adequate prior planning. No one in the small town of about 4,000 residents ever thought that an overflight might come crashing down in its boundary. It can be candidly said from personal observation that, in the initial stages, the Dumfries & Galloway Constabulary, the police authority for Lockerbie, had no accurate or realistic understanding of the scope and severity of the incident, let alone a response plan for the crash of an overflight. The Constabulary moved its response headquarters twice as the incident grew. Even cooperation with outside authorities was unplanned and tense with an uncertain local chain of command. Lessons have been learnt, and the Constabulary today is promoting disaster awareness and planning (Dumfries).

DVI planning is contingent on realistic perceptions. Many people think that they know disasters from Hollywood movies. As Peter Jutro states, "Although virtually no Hollywood blockbuster film is without its errors (it is Hollywood, after all)" (Jutro). The scripts are not totally real and factual to serve as a basis for planning, nor are documentary films made for television or post-incident public relations necessarily accurate

DOI: 10.4324/9781003345367-3

precise. The latter rarely give an accurate and critical assessment of what happened. The choice of events is selective, usually supporting a particular perspective. Devising a DVI plan is best done by consulting with responders who have had practical disaster response experience and can speak on a frank basis.

As the DVI program started at the Israel Police, for example, DVI responders from abroad were invited to give seminars, so they could explain what went right and what went wrong at disasters within their experience. This enabled candid discussion with question and answer. Larger meetings, such as those convened by Interpol, were beneficial to increase understanding, but their scale and public nature prevented most critical exchanges. They did, however, provide networking for follow-up contacts.

From the very beginning, even in planning stages, it must be realized that disaster responders are not super-human when confronted with mass deaths and unpleasant sights. The responders can react similarly to bereaved families, who often display emotions when trying to help identify their deceased loved ones. This psychology must be understood as part of DVI planning and training. A seasoned pathologist retired to his office to recompose himself after seeing the body of a friend. Police are also not immune to psychological factors (Marshall) and at times tend to hide symptoms, since they are considered not to be career enhancing. After one terrorist attack, a trained and experienced police fingerprint technician could not take prints from a deceased whom he had recognized.

Organizations and government agencies have put together DVI manuals and accompanying forms in multiple languages. Perhaps the most common set of forms has been published and distributed by Interpol (Interpol), which established a DVI Standing Committee in the late 1970s.

The establishment of Interpol's DVI Standing Committee can be seen from a broader historical perspective, as part of a general civilization of DVI from military responsibility to general civilian authorities. As DVI moved to be based increasingly on more scientific methods, the differences between military and civilian identification widened. Part of the reason was adapting crime-fighting forensics to DVI.

Professional armies are based on assigned tasks, "dog tags" (ID tags) worn by soldiers, and identification files made specifically in case of the soldier's death in the line of duty, hardly the case with civilians, particularly in open population disasters. Thus, it became increasingly evident that as the gap widened, a purely civilian DVI structure was needed. (A later but parallel development was PTSD, moving from "battle fatigue" to civilian terminology and treatment. See later.)

Other organizations have produced forms and manuals including the Pan American Health Organization (PAHO) and jurisdictions at different levels of government. The PAHO manual has multiple co-sponsors, purporting to be an internationally accepted guide.

In any event, it is pointless to simply adopt a ready-made manual and say, "That's it. Done!" Any manual taken from the shelf must be adapted to a local situation.

Much in on-shelf manuals is repetitive. Sometimes, it is speculative. Other times, it is irrelevant to a local situation. There are differences in approach. Much depends on local capabilities. These are just some of the reasons why manuals must be adapted to local circumstances.

There are differences of opinion and approach in designing a DVI program. There are, to give just one example, those professionals who recommend that a medical examiner visit the scene to obtain an overall understanding of what happened, while other manuals do not feel that this is necessary. It is hard to just follow the book. Rather than blindly following the manual like a check list, it is best to estimate local manpower and leave many questions to a professional's judgment.

DVI planning must be integrated into the overall response protocol. This means assessing manpower, deciding on facilities with options for expansion and storage of bodies, acquisition, and refill of supplies, agreements for supplementary professional and administrative staff, rest areas, communication arrangements to avoid system overload, etc. It is obvious that this is not a quick task. It takes careful work for a disaster that everyone hopes will never happen. That is the source of a common mistake sometimes based on a false premise—avoiding work on a task that may never be put to practical use.

The following chapters describe the DVI information that must be collected. Forms are a key part of DVI planning. Once a DVI plan is devised, forms need to be prepared. DVI information cannot be randomly jotted down on chits of paper or in a notebook. It must be collected in an orderly fashion—on forms prepared in advance that are carefully thought out. In several incidents, master copies of the chosen DVI forms were quickly duplicated in sufficient quantity after a disaster occurred. It is a local decision if forms are to be printed in hardcopy or digitalized. Although DVI experts play a major role in designing (and updating) forms, at least the *ante mortem* (*AM*—data collected from the period when a person was alive) forms are best filled out with the aid of people trained to relate to the bereaved and question them. The Interpol forms, periodically updated, are quite popular.

In theory, one might postulate that, in seemingly local incidents, the choice of any set of professional forms is sufficient. The fallacy of this thinking is that many incidents thought to be "local" can really be international. A prime example is the building collapse in Surfside, Florida (24 June 2021). Although the condominium was residential, it housed many residents and tenants from abroad or with relatives abroad who provided DVI information, not only in English.

The unified use of a standard form simplifies information recording and sorting. Every form has its positive and negative aspects. Preference is often given to the Interpol DVI manual and accompanying forms that are found with the procedures manual. AM information after a disaster is most often collected by police, and the multi-language Interpol forms take that into consideration. Foreign languages are not only needed for data collection from abroad. Many countries, including the United States, have citizens and residents more comfortable with a language other than the national tongue.

Experience has shown that the Interpol AM forms can take up to two hours to complete (Figure 2.1). This has definite advantages to assist the bereaved psychologically by involving him/her in the identification process and collecting a large amount of information in one interview. There are, however, disadvantages. The long form ties up manpower (even when fill-in is administrated by volunteers) and can delay identification. In many cases, the forms require information that is subjective or is not really needed in the specific case. Given these considerations, one country's DVI unit developed a much shorter version of the Interpol form using many of the same questions (translated into the local language) and the same numbering system, just omitting questions less frequently needed. This was done to strike a balance between bereaved involvement and more rapid identification.

Many standard forms also describe clothing worn by a deceased according to Western style. Even in Western countries, forms must be adjusted to

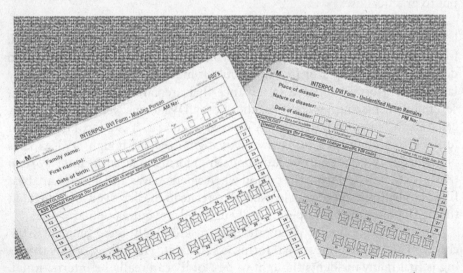

Figure 2.1 Example of the Interpol DVI information forms: AM (left) and PM (right).

include non-Western ethnic dress such as is common in various Arab countries or Oriental and Sub-Continent communities.

There is no intrinsic problem in multiple people separately having filled out *AM* forms regarding the same victim. Although this might seem like unnecessary duplication, this can happen in the pandemonium of a disaster. A side benefit can be the fact that different people remember differently.

If body extrication is moving at a slow pace, filling out abbreviated forms to speed identification might not be the best route to take. Choice of the appropriate version of the forms is a management decision.

In any event, all of these response steps must be integrated into general disaster response plans. For example, when a temporary body examination facility is chosen, communication with the overall incident command center must be arranged in advance, as well as transfer of bodies, release of bodies for burial, etc.

The DVI plan is set. A permanent DVI administrative team is chosen. This is a nucleus—a few people depending on the size of the jurisdiction. Their job will be to make budgetary requests, coordinate with overall disaster responders, select personnel to be on loan from needed disciplines in times of disasters, arrange training, procure and update equipment, etc.

The DVI permanent team must produce a working protocol coordinated with the overall plans approved by the local jurisdiction. Merely copying an existent manual with local adaptations and placing it into a drawer are insufficient to check off, "Done." It must be distributed. It must be read. And, it must be re-read from time to time.

In one airport interview, it took an area manager of a foreign airline ten minutes to find the emergency procedures manual! At first, one might think that, okay, an airline manager is not connected to DVI managers. Wrong! Liaison with an airline after a crash is important for DVI. The station manager and his supervisors must know what services and information the airline is expected to provide. One approach is periodic liaison and coordination with an Airline Operator's Committee (AOC), found at every commercial airport served by regular airlines. A typical AOC has meetings with representatives present from all airlines servicing the airport with scheduled flights.

It is impractical for every town and city under a flight path to be in contact with airlines. They should, however, maintain a contingency plan and working relationship with appropriate civil aviation authorities that will be able to render assistance in times of need.

Modern aviation procedures add certain complications to traditional procedures. Many airlines are not represented at airports that they service. They contract all functions to ground handling companies that almost always service more than one carrier. Code-sharing, a term coined in 1989, means that two or more carriers assign and sell tickets to a flight that is operated by one single carrier. That is to say that the partner airlines need not have any representation at an airfield.

Once planning is set, a team must be assembled. In terms of DVI, prospective members should be screened for physical and psychological issues that might interfere with job performance, not relaying on the assumption that all policemen or all responders are healthy. (In one disaster response a worker dealing with purely bureaucratic paperwork encountered psychological problems and was approved for early retirement several months later.)

Next comes training the team, not only in aspects of the disaster response plan but also in the general characteristics of a disaster so that they understand the milieu in which they will be working. This must include physical and psychological health issues that may be involved and the precautions needed. Although this training does take away potential responders from their routine duties, it is a necessary step in preparing for disaster.

It must be stressed that DVI responders are not just individuals. They are members of a "team." Training must highlight the concept of working together. They must look out for each other, watching for even slight injury to co-workers, stress, physical and psychological exhaustion, or other signs of adverse and problematic reactions. That is inherent in team work.

Other participants in training must be those at various administrative and political officials at all levels. They must have sufficient background to make informed and rapid decisions when disaster strikes. The onset of a disaster requires briefings on the situation on the ground. It is the time to explain neither the mechanics of disaster response nor the background reasons for the pace of work in the field.

Exercises

A popular and necessary approach to disaster planning is to conduct exercises. Mere reading a manual, even "once in a while," is insufficient (although refresher reading is always necessary). Exercises are always essential.

There are two contexts for effective DVI response exercises. One is DVI-specific, exercising the roles and actions of DVI responders. The other is much more general, including DVI in the context of an overall response.

Design a realistic scenario for the disaster, then what? Exercises must be devised at different levels of structure and complexity. When properly formulated, these exercises will teach, test, and identify weak spots.

Many managers like to show success, so they formulate exercises that are designed to succeed. In the eyes of many, it would not be very job-enhancing to have potential responders and trainees fail. Exercises should not be overly complex for the level of the participants, nor should they be too simple. Perhaps it is best to say that exercise should present a challenge. After all, real disasters are anything but routine. Each disaster response is a series of challenges.

One common problem with exercises of all kinds, particularly in large police departments, is trainees having frequent assignment changes. It is a distinct possibility they will be re-assigned before the next exercise or before a real event. Therefore, a schedule of periodic refreshers must be put into effect. This is true at all levels and in all functions. Airline station managers are reassigned. Municipal employees change assignments or retire.

There are different types of exercises held at various stages of disaster planning.

Table Top

One commercial company with a keen understanding of exercises describes the different types of table top exercises in the context of a no pressure and stress-free group activity to develop, learn, and test emergency procedures. The tabletop exercise is a step toward moving from theory to the practical application of operational plan. It identifies problems identification and identifies issues that must be solved or clarified. For example, as bodies are extricated from a collapsed building, which unit should be tasked with photography. This is often in conversational mode. This often generates a constructive discussion promoting clarification of protocols. It often raises procedural questions. How many photographs should be taken? How many hours should a work shift last? Is there psychological oversight of the photographer?

The success of an exercise is not, "Okay. All problems are solved." That might make a nice report to senior management but the opposite is true, "In an active discussion, key problems were identified for refinement and/or resolution. A tabletop exercise is just as it says—tabletop. No equipment is used (perhaps with the exception of a voice recorder for later reference). No one is sent to the field. It incurs little budgetary cost."

Advanced table top exercises are more complex. They can present a multi-faceted situation with responses needed from numerous players in an organization. It can also include representatives from outside organizations needed in a response. For example, a bus skids off a road and overturns in a ravine with a river. Put a clock on the wall, and let's start talking. Who does what? What equipment do we need? Does the bus company have a role? Injured to hospital, but what is the procedure with those officially declared dead? Obviously, a key factor is coordination between organizational participants.

Proper exercises require extensive planning, a key part of which is setting goals and inviting the appropriate participants. Inviting the oversight of an independent and out-of-area critic can be helpful in providing his insight (Preparedex—https://preparedex.com/).

Every exercise should be an opportunity to strengthen cooperation and coordination. Do not say, "Not needed. We work together all the time." Yes, police coordinate with fire on a routine basis, closing off the operational area around a raging fire. That does not mean that fire/traffic have practiced coordinating with DVI as fire fighters periodically douse the overturned bus in the ravine as a precaution to prevent further conflagration as extrication and DVI teams try to work.

Another company has developed a sophisticated, computerized simulation for disaster scenarios. The simulations include detailed mapping of areas, locations of response facilities, and resources ranging from fire stations to ambulance locations to basic equipment. Thus, exercises can be run in a realistic environment.

Multi-agency participation in exercises is necessary, so that DVI can be viewed in its proper context, including testing communication lines (e.g., to search and rescue teams, triage stations). The exercises should include realistic scenarios for body extrication, refrigeration in temporary holding areas, and transfer to a DVI facility of appropriate size.

Body contamination (disease, chemical, and other biological) must also be exercised in a DVI context. This should include hazard identification, DVI team protection, decontamination of deceased and property, etc. This includes fielding of a medical assessment before DVI teams enter the scene. In a terrorist incident involving explosives, entry to the scene should be coordinated with Explosive Ordnance Disposal (EOD) personnel.

Another realistic method for a tabletop exercise is to time responses and reactions with a clock or stopwatch. This brings increased reality to the exercise. Obviously, the clock can be stopped for comments or clarifications.

Field

There is considerable discussion about both the nature and value of DVI field exercises. The primary conclusion is that table-top exercises should precede field exercises. The basic goal of the table-top is to teach procedures to personnel with new assignments and to refresh working rules for veteran employees. With this in place, field exercises can be undertaken. The field exercise should be designed with a realistic scenario after initial training.

A field exercise is a costly stage, putting together the experiences and lessons learnt from smaller "dry" table-top exercises. Often field exercises are filmed and selectively edited, then publicized to show their having taken place. Fine, but all footage should be examined for critical analysis and identification ot weak spots. Lessons learnt are important aspect of any and every exercise.

In many field exercises, investigators have been assigned administrative tasks (e.g., logging in bodies). This seems to be a dubious use of manpower trained in investigations. It might give them a better understanding of the overall body-handling process, but it does nothing to prune their investigative skills or expose them to the problems of identification.

Many exercises tend to deal exclusively with registering and tagging "victims," collecting *AM* data, avoiding such considerations as logistics (water, electricity, air quality, etc.), and work flow.

A common protocol calls for an annual disaster exercise at airports, each year practicing a different aspect of disaster planning. One approach is to dress up victims with visual "injuries" to create a sense of reality. This adds cost to the exercise. There are other questions, such as ignoring internal injury and the proper place to simulate medical triage questions such as medical prioritization of triage and evacuation as well as choice of hospital based on type of injury and hospital capacity.

Airports routinely concentrate on aviation disasters, ideally according to professional requirements on an annual basis. The best procedure is not to repeat the same exercise every year, but rather to vary the scenario, testing different parts of planning. From a DVI perspective, passenger terminal fires and terrorist attacks on areas frequented by passengers before boarding are also fertile areas for airport exercises. Discussions with airport officials should raise the issue of DVI in the exercises. In one exercise, injured "passengers" were evacuated to hospital; at the same time, there had been a theoretical traffic accident. One conclusion from the exercise was that there was confusion as to which patients came from which event. Even for DVI purposes, there must be a separation, although from a medical perspective, treatment priority makes no distinction of the disaster in which a patient was injured.

In designing local jurisdiction drills, it is quite practical to run exercises under an "all hazards" approach and not necessarily for specific hazards. It can be quite difficult to convince some jurisdictions to plan for disaster response, let alone run exercises. "It won't happen here." "FEMA (Federal Emergency Management Agency), or the FBI (Federal Bureau of Investigation) will handle it." Those, or similar agencies in countries abroad might eventually render assistance or even assume responsibility after time, but there is no replacement for immediate local response. Outside response takes time until it starts.

General and later President Dwight Eisenhower is often quoted as saying, "I have always found that plans are useless, but planning is indispensable." The same quote is applicable to DVI. A disaster involving DVI is not just a small incident blown up on a larger scale. Every disaster has its unique problems. There must be planning, but there must be a mind-set to apply basic thinking and experience to new and unforeseen situations. Flexibility is critical. Exercises should help create a disaster mind-set.

Before leaving the subject of exercises, it should be pointed out that not "everything" can be exercised in any one exercise. Goals for each exercise must be set even in the earliest planning stages.

Response to mass disasters is rarely limited to involvement of only one jurisdictional authority. It can be very helpful to conduct exercises jointly with other local jurisdictions and in some cases a national team. This leads into the subject of "players."

DVI and Other Players

3

There are numerous "players" (organizations or formal groups performing a specific function) involved in response to a disaster. DVI is only one (with a caveat) such player. It is not a self-sustaining and independent entity. For DVI to function properly, it must coalesce with other players.

Some players are obvious, such as medical and fire responders. Often, they constitute several "players." If there are two or more ambulance services or fire departments, each is considered a separate player, since each requires its own working and coordination protocol. Not to be forgotten are the scene cleanup and wreckage removal workers fielded at the very end of the response. Each of these functions can have more than one "player." Police responders, even when belonging to the same police department, account for numerous players, since again the various units require their own coordination protocols. Thus, DVI is one or more of the numerous police players. Other police examples are functions such as traffic and various logistics units (e.g., food, drink, portable bathrooms, hygiene supplies, working kits, communication gear, supervision, and site security). If there is more than one DVI team, each is considered a "player." Also not to be forgotten are support functions such as spokesmanship.

In incidents of all types, there are also representatives of the local authority, be it municipality or airport. Then there can be employees of an airline or bus company.

A unique player who should be present particularly in a large response is an invited independent observer, often an academic, to provide an independent, informed, and unbiased evaluation of performance for post-incident evaluation and lessons learnt. This applies to the overall operation and to DVI as well.

As has been noted several times, DVI must be integrated into the entire overall picture. Teams in a large incident often have to be brought in from afar. This means a gradual increase in the number of players and issuing of work assignments and instructions.

The DVI process is dependent upon a proper information flow and a wide variety of players, not all of whom are DVI specialists (Figure 3.1). First the process works with interactions in the field, and then it concentrates on concrete identification procedures (Figure 3.2).

DOI: 10.4324/9781003345367-4

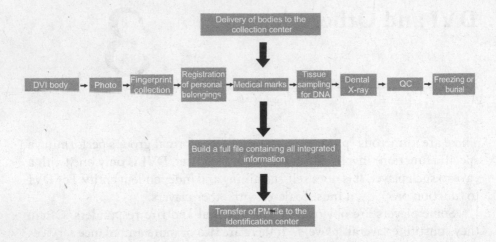

Figure 3.1 Process line for the preparation of PM DVI file.

Source: Information collected from two bodies in parallel lines.

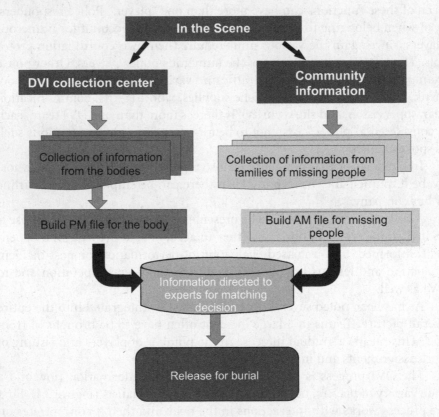

Figure 3.2 DVI identification process which include collection of information from the reported missing person and collection of information from the body.

For DVI responders, the initial notification received usually means rapid response to an unclear situation even though it is often said that the dead "can wait." These initial responders should take with them starting equipment that should be kept ready for emergency, to be supplemented by additional supplies after incident size assessment.

In many ways, DVI cannot be divorced from scene photography. It is always important to record the location in which a body and property are found (detailed later). It is insufficient to make only individual records. Bodies must always be photographed in the greater context of the overall incident. In an air crash, for example, exact location can be a strong help in associating family members having sat together and reconstructing the seating plan, recognizing that there can be changes after boarding or in-flight. In a bus bombing, as in an air crash, people sitting together can be associated with each other or random, but there is rarely a seating assignment particularly in urban bus lines.

Not related to DVI, seating and injuries can provide evidence of the location of an explosive. Seating, however, can also help DVI as a suggestion of familial, group, business, or friendship relationships.

When bodies are moved before photography for purposes of saving lives or site safety, interviews should be conducted to determine initial body location.

From these varied examples, it can be seen that overall site coordination is essential. No response function, i.e., no "player," is absolutely independent.

The guiding rule of DVI is that "identification is the positive comparison of *ante mortem* and *post mortem* (*PM*—data collected from a cadaver) information of sufficient importance." Some information is significant; other information is not significant for positive identification, but it can be important for elimination. "He was short." "She had jet black hair." These are examples of features that are insignificant as the basis of an identification in a large population, but they can be used for exclusion. If a missing male person was tall, all short males and all females can be excluded as possibilities for identification. Of course, short and tall can be subjective judgments, and allowances should be taken for such.

As years of experience have taught, the definition of identification is seemingly straight-forward, but practical application renders it unabatedly and excessively simplistic. Cultural norms can be an important element. Significance can depend on population size. DVI standards remain the same, but working conditions often open up procedural questions. What is considered "of sufficient importance?" There are cultural considerations. In certain societies, having a beard or pierced nose is more common than not.

In discussing DVI, a cardinal rule is that one must remember the working atmosphere is one of a disaster and not a traffic accident involving one or two fatalities. Mass disasters involve public pressure, media coverage, sometimes political interference, and by definition an overload stretching routine capabilities.

DVI is not a task that can be properly completed in the field in open spaces. Proper facilities are needed. Most day-to-day forensic working spaces are designed to accommodate a work load much less than that in a disaster. How can overload of facilities be minimalized? Experience has shown several answers.

- After the Air Inter Flight 148 air crash (20 January 1992, Airbus flight from Lyons, France crashed in the Vosges Mountains near Mont Sainte-Odile, while preparing to land at Strasbourg), refrigerated tents were erected for storage, and bodies were brought to the forensic center only in stages. All 87 people lost their lives. Nine others survived freezing winter temperatures, as responders spent long hours searching for the wreckage in the mountainous terrain.
- Following a helicopter crash in the Israel Air Force (4 February 1997, two transport helicopters collided in mid-air, killing all 73 Israeli military personnel onboard), more than 70 bodies were brought to a large but no longer used funeral facility where most *PM* examinations were conducted. It was realized that certain heavy equipment could not be brought, and some victims still had to be transferred to the Institute of Forensic Medicine. At least the funeral facility reduced the burden on the forensic institute but not on its professional staff.

If a temporary facility is used, it should be built for crowd control and contain water, bathrooms, electricity, etc., such as a professional sports stadium.

As odd as this may sound, the DVI goal should be set even at an initial stage. This will run through the entire operation. The Twin Towers 9/11 disaster covered 64,500 m^2 with 18 million tons of rubble and human remains almost 44 meters deep. It took 3 months to extinguish the last fires and almost 9 months to clear debris. In total, 22,000 bodies and fragments of the 2,753 victims were found. Only after almost six years did the New York City Medical Examiner's Office announce having achieved identification of 1,133 victims (several more have been identified since). Forty-one percent of the total remained unidentified.

There is a clear reason why the identification goal for each incident must be set at the very onset of the operation. There is a major difference between identifying all remains, identifying at least one part of every victim, and identifying a part of a victim's body without which life cannot be sustained. A corollary to this question is the subject of co-mingled body parts.

Often a balance must be met in setting an identification policy. On the one hand, a disaster may be caused by a criminal act and should be treated as a crime scene even in dealing with fatalities. On the other hand, the mere scope of the disaster, traffic jams, and political implications can preclude time consuming actions. If there is a guiding principle, it is that professionalism should never be compromised at the expense of expedience. Fine to be said, but sometimes difficult to implement!

Public Inquiries Center

4

Many times, it is not clear who was involved in a disaster. Airplane manifests are more or less accurate, but earthquakes are quite different. An important part of disaster victim identification is establishing a list of missing persons, i.e., possible victims to be identified. One aspect of constructing missing person lists is establishing an information center to which people can call and inquire about persons possibly connected to the disaster.

People worry about their families and friends. Experience has shown that most calls are unconnected to the incident, but relevant inquiries provide needed follow-up information. Although this has important ramifications for DVI, the Center is not staffed by DVI personnel. Specific staffing is very often determined by the type of incident involved. Airlines and large municipalities often supply personnel with language skills; small bus companies and villages rarely do. Centers often require 24/7 operation in their initial stages. There should be an overall manager, shift managers, and staff trained in disaster response including psychology issues and DVI.

In any event, contact information (telephone, email, and social media) needed to operate the center should be prepared in advance by disaster response officials and then activated immediately after initial reports of a disaster. The Center can never be opened *too* early. There will be a flood of access attempts, and busy lines only heighten caller apprehension. All types of contact (telephone, digital, and fax) should be adequately staffed for rapid response. When received, inquiries all must be sorted for probability and thereby prioritized for handling. A lexicon of terms should be prepared in advance to avoid misunderstandings and uniformity of language.

Staffing poses interesting questions. Initial preparations for the Boston Marathon anticipated some 80 telephone calls. Some 8,600 inquiries were received in the first 24 hours after disaster struck (DePaolo, Frank). This means technological preparation for network expansion and quick personnel call out even during non-working hours or holidays.

One method to prune out irrelevant calls early in the process is to precede contact with a human responder with a recorded statement containing basic details of the incident: for example, "If you are calling in regard to AB Flight 123 that departed City on 00 January at 0000" and "If you are calling in regard to the fire at 123 Main Street, Centerville on 00 February at 1200."

DOI: 10.4324/9781003345367-5

Only a portion of the inquiries received at an information center will eventually require DVI handling. If there hopefully are survivors, those cases will be referred to other sources for very different handling. Survivors can be categorized thusly:

- Not injured.
- Light injury. Treated at the scene.
- Light injury. Treated at hospital and released.
- Injury requiring hospitalization.
- Severe injury and cannot communicate effectively.

Reports of all survivors should be transferred from the Public Inquiries Center to an overall Information Center, so that a list of all involved can be created. Obviously, this includes even those treated at the scene and quickly released. This will be important in incident investigation, clarifying the status of missing persons, and thus also DVI.

In countless disasters, there have been numerous inquiries about people who were, happily, not at all involved in the incident. It is common that in cases in which the person in question is finally located, the missing person report will not be canceled by the person making the notification. A common phenomenon is that people are so overjoyed to find a missing person sound and well that they neglect to notify authorities. A true example is a boy who was reported missing from the area of a disaster and could not be reached by his family; he was on a hiking adventure of several days. Only in a follow-up call to the family were authorities able to cancel the missing person notification.

It is prudent to grade the probability of missing person reports, so that initial attention can be paid to those that seem most probable. Evaluations can be updated as an incident progresses.

Since DVI is an important recipient of the information collected, identification needs must be taken into consideration even at an early stage of contact. Information collection forms should be set in place as an advance preparation so that nothing is forgotten in the initial information collection stage.

Open and Closed Populations

The Public Inquiries Center is just one tool to ascertain who are the potential victims in a disaster. This goes well beyond the specific interests of DVI. There are many other players and functions involved.

Different disasters present different population challenges. An airplane that crashes, for example, always has a passenger manifest. Sometimes the manifest is accurate, sometimes not. A chartered helicopter that started from Herzliya, Israel, on its way to Masada crashed on a farm in the Negev (25 November 1993). It had five people aboard—a Chinese woman, a Chinese man, and three Israelis. This was a "closed population" with a relatively simple identification needing verification but not intensive investigation.

There are, of course, populations that are theoretically closed, but not hermetically so. The passenger lists for the Titanic (sunk in the North Atlantic Ocean on 15 April 1912) posed fewer problems in first and second classes, but there was a literal free-for-all or anything-goes in third class, where the estimated number of passengers has varied by more than 100, and now after more than 100 years later even the number of third-class passengers is still uncertain. Clearly, the latter passage was an open population with only a partially reliable passenger list.

The crash of El Al cargo flight 1862 (4 October 1992) into two residential buildings in the Bijlmermeer neighborhood of Amsterdam presents two different populations. Those aboard the flight were a "closed population" (three male crew members and a non-paying female passenger), but persons in the residential buildings were a type of "open population." Who was at home? Were there guests? Were there people who claimed to be there for insurance purposes? (One supposed "victim" of 9/11 "buried in the rubble" called for help from a cellphone, as he sat comfortably far away in Newark, New Jersey.) The neighborhood had a high crime rate, a consequence of which was that many claims of involvement were viewed with initial suspicion.

Not to be forgotten, even in standard air crashes not all passenger lists are accurate or honest. Terrorists, for example, have sometime used bogus passports to obscure their true identity when boarding a flight. This is true not only on the way to their mission but also in prior planning stages.

There are numerous cases of illegal immigrants or criminals traveling under assumed names or falsified/stolen identification papers, thus complicating subsequent DVI.

The sinking of illegal migrant ships crossing the Mediterranean Sea or the English Channel is particularly problematic for DVI purposes. A vessel carrying 29 passengers (27 dead, 2 survivors) left from France to England on 24 November 2021. The clandestine nature of the voyage meant no passenger list. In many cases, even close family were not aware of the trip. Pictures of possible victims were circulated, but bloating from the water complicated even tentative identification. The passengers also came from Third World countries, not necessarily renowned for detailed record keeping, so reliable AM data became difficult to obtain.

The sinking of a migrant ship in the Mediterranean Sea on 3 October 2013 is another example. One hundred and fifty-five passengers survived, but 366 perished. Not all bodies were recovered, and of those found, many were not identified. A major problem was that many were refugees from countries at war or experiencing situations in which ruling forces could not be contacted to obtain *AM* information.

Defining the distance covered by a disaster is key in establishing the potential population in question. A plane crash is not as simple as it might seem. Pan Am 103 flight (21 December 1988) fell primarily in and around Lockerbie, but not exclusively so. A wide search was initiated to find parts of the plane and possible victims. Pieces of the aircraft were found in an area of 200 km². Eleven residents of a Lockerbie neighborhood, Sherwood Crescent, lost their lives as parts of the plane descended onto their houses, some of which were destroyed by fire starting with unused aviation fuel. Fortunately, no other parts caused death on the ground. Determining the population in the disaster was not immediate, as one might think.

The 6.9 Richter Scale San Francisco earthquake on 17 October 1989 presented a totally different "open population" scenario. A key element of the response with DVI ramifications was to define the area of possible damage serious enough to merit search for those trapped in debris or otherwise incapable of calling for help. Reports of missing persons were numerous in a totally "open population" situation.

DVI Equipment 5

It is important to document details of a disaster site for numerous reasons in addition to DVI. The exact location of bodies can be important. The various players in a response photograph the disaster for their own objectives. DVI is no different.

The digital era has made a major change in our lives. In terms of disaster victim identification, it has literally redefied scene documentation. Film no longer has to be stored for potential use, always watching expiration dates and refreshing supplies. In the same vein, nor does a police technician need to worry about exhausting a 36-frame roll, nor waiting for a laboratory to develop the film and make prints. All is on-the-spot.

The digital era has also meant rapid transmission of documents and information. Fax machines are ubiquitous, as are iPhones that can send and receive material even internationally. Senior policy managers can view aspects of a disaster and make decisions from afar. That is not to say that they can replace on-site managers. Rather, they can assess reports simultaneously from more than one location to acquire a broader understanding of the overall situation and general needs.

Smart phones have had an additional impact on identification. Today a large part of the general population in essence walks around with a camera in a telephone. It is increasingly common for passersby to photograph disasters. Call their motives curiosity or other, the stills and videos can provide significant information for DVI as well as general incident reconstruction.

An interesting application of digital photography is to overlay disaster incidents on local geography ("photo-shopping") as an aid in response planning and exercises to increase realism. These changes have brought a literal evolution to disaster response. There still are, however, standard needs.

The time to acquire equipment for disaster response is long before a disaster takes place. When a disaster occurs, it is not the time for a hurried shopping trip. Take what is already prepared, and, "Go to the scene!"

The last sentence is simplistic. "Go to the scene!" How? What about bringing equipment? For DVI there is no justification to break traffic rules and travel through stop signs and red lights. That is reserved for an ambulance and fire as well as emergency police functions. DVI deals with the dead. DVI responders can travel safely. In any case, it is best not to clutter a scene

DOI: 10.4324/9781003345367-6

while critical life-saving activity is underway. If any exception is to be made, it is only for those DVI technicians dealing with site documentation and photography as part of their assignments.

There are two types of equipment needed for DVI aspects of disaster response: (1) personal and (2) group or team. There is one cardinal rule that governs both types of equipment. It must be disinfected at appropriate times whenever there is the slightest chance of contamination.

Personal Equipment

In an average situation, each DVI police field technician has his own routine equipment for lifting latent fingerprints, photography, etc. This is designed for a typical crime scene, be it a murder, house break-in, or other crime that occurs in the course of his ordinary work. In a disaster scenario, this is only a starter. Much more is needed.

It is axiomatic that every technician be adequately protected before he enters a disaster site. The health dangers go well beyond the average crime scene. Personal protective equipment (PPE) can be needed (Makwana). That means that full body covering may be required—scalp, body, nose/mouth, and foot coverings as well as gloves. This must take into account coverings appropriate not only to the scene but also for the prevailing weather. For example, on a hot summer day, there must be coverings that "breathe" in contrast to provisions for winter cold, not to speak of rain.

Gloves are not a simple issue. If one must deal with sharp edges as in a typical aviation crash or bus bombing, stronger gloves are needed, still allowing finger dexterity. Kevlar gloves are a common solution, but they are not an absolute protection. Care against puncture is still required.

Gloves for specifically for a DVI technician touching human remains are usually nitrile or latex. These gloves adhere to the hand. This means fine dexterity if the proper size is worn. Thus, gloves should also be available in different sizes. They should be disposed in a special container after use with a corpse or body parts. Particularly if there are open wounds or fluids coming from a body, it is prudent to assume the possibility of infection and take appropriate precautions (i.e., PPE). There are DVI technicians (and even pathologists) who prefer thicker cloves to distance themselves psychologically from "touching" and feeling a cadaver (Cohen).

A word of caution is in order. Allergic reactions to latex and nitrile are known phenomena—latex much more so than nitrile. Responders should be aware of their skin sensitivities in an initial pre-incident screening procedure before assignment. (Obviously, there are on-the-spot passer-by responders not undergoing any pre-incident selection or training.)

Many nitrile and latex gloves have an expiration date that is important and must not be ignored. When wearing gloves, one should be careful not to touch exposed parts of one's own body, such as forehead, eyes, and nose. These gloves should be discarded immediately if cut, punctured, or cracked. When disposing of PPE, one should be careful not to contaminate regular clothing and place the PPE items into a special container, not standard garbage. Hands should be washed with a disinfectant consisting of at least 60% alcohol.

A representative of the Hercules Company based in Yavneh, Israel, recommends nitrile as a standard, but notes that there are variations in size and quality amongst manufacturers (most often in the Far East). A way to test quality is to stretch the glove, determining that it does not break or tear easily.

Nitrile gloves are made for different purposes. For standard DVI, a common (universal) glove is usually sufficient. Medical (non-sterile) and surgical (sterile) grades are not necessary. Latex gloves are significantly more expensive.

Foot coverings pose a similar issue, since stepping on a rough edge requires stronger foot protection. That means boots, preferably with a readily disposable throw-away covering.

There is a stereotype picture of a technician dressed in a white disposable gown. The image is very misleading. A technician needs to have his hands free and equipment to work. When dressed in a disposable gown, there is limited possibility for pockets. Even when there is a pocket, it may be too flimsy for a heavy item. One solution is to wear an equipment vest, changeable as needed. If the scene does not require medical protective gear (only after a professional medical assessment), trousers with numerous pockets can be very useful.

A helmet with a light mounted on it is a practical measure to keep hands free, not only for working at night.

Covid-19 has been a modern concern. It is unknown how long the virus remains alive in a deceased person and can still infect (Dijkhuizen), but much is unknown. The disease is apparently excreted from body openings such as nose, mouth, and skin pores. There is little reliable data as to the lifetime of infectious cells *post mortem*. A cautious recommendation is to take into consideration possible infectious risks from all possible Covid-19 corpses (Gabbrielli).

Covid-19 is spread primarily in the air; hence, masks provide significant (but not total) protection.

There always are extreme examples that contradict standard procedures. The Twin Towers Disaster (WTC on 9/11) is one such event. Over 7% of fire responders reportedly suffered from various injuries related not only to fire but also to dust, particulates, noxious gases, chemicals, and fibers. Many members were injured on the day of the disaster or felt ill in the following days. DVI is not an immediate response. It can wait until a site is declared safe to enter and any additional protective gear can be provided based on an assessment of any unique circumstances or risks. One example is the use of goggles in the event of possible eye irritants.

Group Equipment

The location of all bodies and property must be marked and photographed before moving (recognizing the necessity of life-saving measures). This means pre-prepared numbers preferably lit or glowing in the dark and weighted so as not to fly away in the wind. A complimentary method is to attach a bracelet when possible. Technicians should also be given forms to record their actions.

Property should not automatically be associated with a body unless it is physically held by a deceased or in his/her pockets. (On 6 April 1992, a bomb exploded in Afula, Israel. The driver was amongst the 8 fatal victims. His body was found with him holding money in his hand, obviously as part of a fare transaction.) Even a woman's handbag near a body should be given a separate number with its location noted and photographed.

There must be bags, preferably with seals and of various sizes and weights to collect personal property. Property can be of monetary value, and should be guarded properly though all stages of handling using agreed upon procedures (Amar). Chain of evidence for all property should be carefully maintained.

Incident Photography

Photography by passersby can help, but it is neither professional nor necessarily complete. One of the most famous passers-by films is that of Abraham Zapruder (1905–1970, a clothing manufacturer), who by chance caught the John F. Kennedy assassination on an 8-mm Bell & Howell camera. It is what the citizen sees, what he decides to record, and what he succeeds to capture. News organizations also photograph, but their access to the disaster is also restricted, particularly after the site is organized and cordoned off by uniformed responders. There are usually various official "players" who record the scene. All of these efforts do not replace DVI photography. Its aim is very specific and should be done by an identification technician using cameras with capability for both video and stills. Sometimes the equipment (including lighting) is part of a technician's standard working pack, sometimes not. This should be taken into consideration in planning equipment.

Ideally, bodies should be photographed twice, once as quickly after the disaster as possible when the scene is relatively untouched, then after numbers have been assigned to each cadaver and nearby property. The procedure is not redundant, since life-saving measures may disrupt proper photography. All photography is best from different angles to maximize the capture of as much detail as possible.

Too often life-saving measures are thought of as only medical rescue. There are disasters in which explosive ordnance teams, medical experts, and/ or structural engineers are needed to declare a disaster site safe for entry to prevent further casualties. That can be as important as standard medical treatment. In many cases, a fire department periodically douses an area to prevent conflagration.

In deciding on priorities, it should be remembered that bodies begin to decompose 24 to 48 hours after death (not just after body discovery), particularly in warmer climates (Fischer). This includes not only internal organs but also external aspects such as facial features.

Equipment Logistics

Usually, responders can drive somewhat near the scene of a disaster, but they cannot drive up right next to the site and unload equipment. Unloading must take into consideration safety and congestion, meaning that equipment must be reasonably portable. In urban congested scenarios, it is impractical to bring equipment even 1 km by motor vehicle. Experience has shown that portable carriers with wheels were needed.

All initial equipment is just that—initial—to allow technicians to begin work. A professional assessment of specific equipment needs is possible only after technicians arrive. As a response progresses, there usually are requests for resupply. Therefore, backup is needed for logistical support where equipment is stored. If the disaster is unexpectedly very large, there should be a list of suppliers and emergency off-hours contact numbers readily available. Relying on equipment resupply from neighboring jurisdictions is not necessarily reliable, since their DVI team may already have been asked to be sent to the disaster.

Lighting

Overall lighting of a disaster site is critical, sometimes not only at night, but that is the responsibility of the site management, not DVI. There are, however, the needs of scene documentation personnel.

Perhaps the most obvious need is to free the hands of workers as much as possible for work connected to documentation and eventual identification. A practical solution is wearing a helmet equipped with a flash light, as noted earlier. That is not to say that a hand-held flashlight might not also be needed at times, but a helmet with light minimizes frees the hands. (Needless to say, battery expiration should always be checked as part of routine planning, and spare batteries should always be on hand.)

Not only does the worker need lighting for his work. It has also been useful to place lit markers next to bodies before their removal, so they can be readily found at night (Amar).

When Disaster Strikes

Facing Disaster 6

Although this book highlights the role of DVI, it must be remembered that DVI is only one part of disaster response. The entire mechanism must function properly, since different parts are often dependent on each other. So is it with initial reporting.

In many disasters, initial reports are received on emergency phone numbers such as the North American 911 or European 112. It must be remembered that the callers are not professional responders. They are ordinary citizens, often highly emotional, often overwhelmed psychologically by what they have seen. Initial reports can be under-estimated or over-exaggerated, but the report should trigger police, ambulance, and/or fire response.

What should be dispatched to the scene based on these reports? In many cases, over-reaction is better than under-reaction. Sixty ambulances responded to a 30 November 2021 shooting at an Oxford, Michigan high school leaving 4 dead and 7 requiring hospitalization. Better more responders than fewer.

One rule is basic. It is the responsibility of the first *professional* responder on scene to give a realistic assessment of the scope of the disaster, if known. Obviously, the Oxford situation was a live incident with no way to know with a degree of certainty the situation inside the school. There are, however, other cases. In practical terms, this means that after a disaster such as an air crash, train accident, or bus bombing the first person on scene should report and not start saving lives. In the end, accurate reporting will save more lives, since appropriate and sufficient teams can be sent. That does not mean counting injured and dead. A serious initial estimation of response personnel needed and resources required is an estimate and not an exact head count.

Accurate assessment also has its implications for DVI as well as treating medical issues. Not all DVI response must be immediate. Assessment provides notice. It is recommended on the one hand that scene documentation be done as early as possible. It is helpful not only to DVI but also to other functions. Saving lives obviously takes precedence over identification of the deceased. A good assessment of the situation allows lead time to decide what equipment and its quantity, subject to later adjustment and replenishing, will be sent to the disaster site.

DOI: 10.4324/9781003345367-8

Some disasters involve unique aspects, such as unusual health and safety issues that require special protective measures or equipment for especially dangerous terrain. In these cases, all DVI (and other) teams should be briefed before entering the site.

It is important to understand the nature of various types of disasters, since their character and typical injuries can affect DVI.

Earthquake

An earthquake is generated by a sudden movement of tectonic plates under the earth's surface. Earthquakes cannot be predicted to the level of exact location, hour, day, or even year. There are, however, indications of general probability. "Faults" are the intersection of two or more plates. A mapping of plate intersections is why certain areas have been more prone to earthquakes than others (Dzeboev).

Even if there has been no recorded earthquake in a particular area, there is no guarantee that there will not be a quake at some time.

There are earthquakes occurring every day, but the vast majority are felt only by instrumentation. Only the stronger intensity quakes interest the general public. There are two commonly used methods to measure the intensity or "seriousness" of an earthquake.

The Richter Scale was developed by Charles Richter (1900–1985) in 1935, although it has since been modified. What is today commonly called the Richter scale is, in fact, the Moment Magnitude Scale. The scale classifies the magnitude of an earthquake or the amount of energy released.

The Mercalli Scale was developed by Giuseppe Mercalli (1850–1914) in 1902, and it also has been modified since then. The Mercalli Scale measures the effects of an earthquake at a given location (more relevant to the general public). (There are numerous other scales, either historical or professional but not widely used in popular circles.)

All too often intense earthquakes bring devastation, injury, and death, but that is not always the case. Location is a critical factor. An earthquake in Los Angeles has more consequences than even a stronger event in the Arctic Circle. Also of influence are factors such as depth, type of soil, and building codes. For DVI purposes even high scale numbers on either scale are not necessarily significant. When there are fatalities, the dead have to be identified.

There are usually some rapid identifications, often accompanied in the media by moving descriptions of the life of the deceased and the loss to his family. Identification, however, can be a long and time-consuming process, particularly after a serious earthquake. Delay in locating bodies obviously means delay in identification, a traumatic period for next-of-kin.

Earthquakes often cause other types of disasters. The ground trembling can be a trigger for further damage, essentially a domino effect. The initial earthquake can be a harbinger of what is to come, since it is not necessarily the cause of all damage or death. Aftershocks can also be deadly. The San Francisco/Loma Prieta earthquake of 1989 was 6.9 on the Richter Scale, but there were significant aftershocks. A magnitude 5.2 aftershock occurred approximately 2.5 minutes after the main shock. In the week following Loma Prieta, there were 20 aftershocks measuring a magnitude 4.0 or greater, as well as more than 300 of magnitude 2.5 or greater, the latter hardly felt and causing no damage. There were also hundreds of even weaker trembling not strong enough to be perceived without instrumentation.

Common problems in earthquakes are gas pipe breaks, downed electrical lines, and fires. There can also be structural damage to buildings, landslides, and tsunamis. Response is often delayed due to damage to roads, bridges, and tunnels. Life-saving efforts can also be hampered until roads are passable, and an area is rendered safe.

Building damage or collapse are only stereotyped examples of destruction causing death following an earthquake. Following the San Francisco Earthquake of 18 April 1906, most fatalities were due to fire. There are other effects of earthquakes. Just to remind, earthquakes are known to cause tsunamis, a recent example of which was in the Indian Ocean Tsunami of 26 December 2004. Most serious tsunamis follow an earthquake of at least 7.6 on the Richter scale, and they are felt at large distances. On 1 April 1946, for example, an 8.6 Richter earthquake in the Aleutian subduction zone had effects in Hawaii, where 173 people perished.

There are also mudslides, flooding, and land liquefaction. The bottom line is that body extrication can be a lengthy procedure, and the physical condition of the dead does not always allow for rapid identification, even when *ante mortem* records are available. Causes of death can range from suffocation to crushing to fire.

Given this background, it is a mistake to plan "earthquake DVI" as an isolated activity that can be wrapped up in a matter of days or weeks. If one counts time in terms of days or weeks, that can be a description of the efforts to extricate victims—first the living, then the dead (Rom). An ironic fact is that extrication can be more rapid in underdeveloped areas, where buildings that have collapsed are not sophisticated. It is easier to recover a body from under a wooden shack than in the rubble of a multi-floor concrete housing project.

As in all jobs, it is essential to set objectives before starting to work. Extrication or body retrieval is not necessarily self-understood. Of course, one wants to recover all bodies and body parts, but where does the effort end? In Jewish law, literally everything must be collected from the scene,

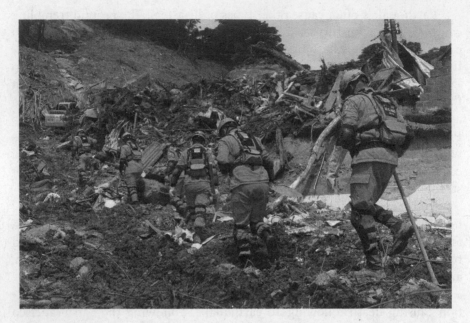

Figure 6.1 Often, scenes of mass casualties require teams to search for body parts and collect DVI remains and belongings that may help in DVI identification.

Source: www.shutterstock.com

including small pieces of flesh and blood, but that is not a DVI objective. DVI is identification—not site cleanup, not burial, not cremation. Once a victim is identified (Figure 6.1), the question of missing body parts and possible later association (reconstitution) with the deceased involves an administrative decision regarding when to bury or cremate.

Air Crash

According to the U.S. Aviation Disaster Family Assistance Act (Appendix F), DVI after an aviation disaster in the United States is the responsibility of the "local medical examiner or coroner," who has the authority to request outside assistance. The identification must be "thorough, deliberate, and based on proven scientific methods." This basic approach has also been adopted by ICAO.

Air crashes do not necessarily occur at the departing or destination airports. Those airports are set up for crashes with the size of airplanes using the airfield. An aircraft in emergency, however, can land at an "alternate airport." That is to say an airport *en route* that is designated as appropriate to accept emergency landings. A small rural air field cannot accept a jumbo jet, not only because of the size of the landing strip but also because it is ill equipped to offer emergency fire and rescue services on a large enough scale.

There is a significant difference between an alternate airport for emergency and a diversion landing. The latter can be for reasons such as bad weather, a passenger taken seriously ill, or as a precautionary measure due to one of many technical problems.

Lockerbie is only one of many modern crashes that did not take place at an airport. Swissair 111 on 2 September 1998 is an example of a plane lost at sea, near Peggy's Cove, Nova Scotia. Air New Zealand Flight 901 crashed into Mount Erebus in Antarctica on 28 November 1979, far from any quick response. In other words, an air crash can take place literally anywhere. In each scenario, there are different implications for DVI. Part of emergency planning is to take into consideration non-scheduled crises not necessarily during normal working hours.

There are several causes of air crash, and in all of them the crash can be fatal. Pilot error, mechanical failure, terror bombing, major weather event, design defect, and air traffic control error are all possibilities. In 2020, birds flew into a Canadian military flight and caused a fatal crash. In the 1990s, Alia Airlines (now Royal Jordanian) suspended operations to Lagos, Nigeria as a precautionary measure due to potholes in the runway.

The cause with a significant implication for DVI is loss of fuel. The crash of Avianca 052 (25 January 1990) at Cove Neck, NY, was not accompanied by any fire upon impact, a preliminary indication of fuel shortage as the cause of the crash. This means a lower chance of conflagration and fewer if any burnt bodies. (There are flammable materials onboard aircraft in addition to fuel, but not in extremely large quantity. Some fires after aircraft crash are due to flammable materials on the ground.)

There is a crash report of the National Transportation Safety Board (NTSB) for the crash of Air Canada Flight 797 on 2 June 1983. Blood samples were taken from the 18 surviving and 23 deceased passengers, and the sample were analyzed by the FAA's Civil Aeromedical Institute, Oklahoma City, Oklahoma, for carbon monoxide, cyanide, fluorides, and ethyl alcohol. Significantly,

> The [hydrogen] cyanide levels found in the blood samples of the deceased ranged from a low of 0.8 to a high of 5.12 micrograms/ml; the toxic level for cyanide in the blood at which incapacitation occurs is between 0.5 and 0.7 micrograms/ml.

This indicates that fatalities were alive on impact and probably died from inhalation.

Hydrogen cyanide is not just an irritant. It is hazardous.

> The main immediately hazardous gas occurring in cabin fires, in addition to Carbon Monoxide . . . is Hydrogen Cyanide. This is produced

during combustion of wool, silk and many nitrogen-containing syn-
thetics, so is almost guaranteed to occur. . . . However, the more sub-
tle effect of the two main toxic gases produced in aircraft cabin fires,
Carbon Monoxide and Hydrogen Cyanide, is physical incapacitation;
this has often been shown to have prevented successful evacuation
from post-crash fires.

(SKYbrary)

Chaturvedi and Sanders (Chaturvedi) report that there were 95 fire-related
civil passenger aircraft accidents worldwide over a 26 year period, claiming
approximately 2400 lives. Between 1985 and 1991, about 16% (32 accidents) of
all U.S. transport aircraft accidents involved fire and 22% (140 fatalities) of the
deaths in these accidents resulted from fire/smoke toxicity.

This raises the issue of contamination of responders (including DVI) and
appropriate protective gear, not exclusively from dangerous cargo but also
from the cabin upon entering the aircraft.

Building Collapse, Bombings, and Explosions

Some building collapses are the result of factors such as faulty design, sub-
standard building materials, poor construction methods, weak foundation,
or under the forces of natural events such as hurricanes, tornadoes, cyclones,
and earthquakes. Typical signs of problems are cracks in walls, swelling
particularly of support pillars, or paint separating from steel girders, but
sometimes structural phenomena are insufficient indicators, and structural
damage can go unrecognized for extended periods of time. The leaning of the
Millenium Tower in San Francisco is an example of mistaken estimation of
bedrock, and concerted efforts to prevent collapse and ensuing disaster.

During 1951–1952, there were three air crashes in Elizabeth, New Jersey,
a city in a typical landing or takeoff path from Newark Airport's then-North
Terminal. In one of the crashes, debris fell on a local school. No structural
problems were noted at the time, the school continued to operate, and the
incident was forgotten with the passage of time. Only on a weekend in the late
1990s did the roof of the school suddenly collapse, apparently as a result of
the air crash more than 40 years previously. For the record there were numerous fatalities in those 1950s crashes, but professional DVI by forensic means
was still in its infancy, although there were some identifications based on
dentistry. In a more recent tour of the neighborhoods in which the planes fell,
one can see house out-of-period (built later) in place of buildings that had to
be condemned after the crashes.

Other reasons for collapse are intentional, such as after bombing as in
case of the Federal Building in Oklahoma City on 1 April 1995 or other acts

such as the airplane attacks on 9/11. In many incidents, there are implications for DVI.

Linguistically there is a common mistake. Very often people think that implosion and explosion are synonyms. There is a difference that can be critical in locating bodies for victim identification. Explosions are caused by a direct force that releases energy from within a structure that explodes outwards. An implosion is caused by an external force making a structure to implode inward on itself. This difference means a building can collapse, reversing the order of floors (top floor on the bottom) depending on numerous factors. It can be important to have an appropriate expert explain the consequences of a specific bombing. This can explain the location of bodies, important for DVI.

The U.S. Department of Justice through its National Institute of Justice has published an in-depth manual for dealing with a bombing incident (NIJ), including stress in interviewing witnesses and survivors to reconstruct what happened as the incident unfolded. When fatalities are involved, these questions should also involve queries needed for DVI purpose.

Bombings Not in Buildings

It is essential to render an area safe after a bombing, but this can be very different from a fuel spillage or road accident with a truck carrying hazardous materials. Simultaneous and sequential bombings have been known in terrorist incidents. A simultaneous terrorist attack happened in Jerusalem's Machane Yehudah Market on 30 July 1997 at 1:15 in the afternoon. Two suicide bombers carried bags containing explosives and shrapnel. The terrorists set off bombs 45 meters (150 feet) apart simultaneously, killing 16 civilians. From a DVI perspective, it is important not to confuse the victims from each group of fatalities, since proximity to each other may assist in establishing relationships, and hence aid in identification.

A sequential bombing is different. In such a case, one bomb is set off, then after an interval a second bomb is detonated, usually where terrorists estimate the area in which a crowd will be gathering. An example is Zion Square in Jerusalem on 4 September 1997, as three Hamas suicide bombers detonated bombs one after another, killing eight persons. Again, from a DVI perspective, it is important not to confuse the victims from each group of fatalities.

Bus bombings are very different. There are different motives and a different operational response. The goals tend to be three—inflicting injury and death to passengers, disrupting normal routines particularly in busy urban areas, and publicizing the cause of the bombers. As to the latter, the publicity involved in a large event tends to revolve around death and destruction, rather than the terrorist's specific political cause, but that meets the terrorists' goal to instill fear in the populace.

A major difference from a bomb in a building is that in a bus or in an open area body extrication can often be completed in a relatively shorter time. It is hard to cite a case of multiple bombs on a bus; the common *modus operandi* is an abandoned package or a single suicide bomber. Relatively rapid body extrication does not simplify victim identification. In these cases, one is generally talking about a decidedly open population. Chartered busses have not been targeted with onboard bombs, since any stranger is quickly identified as such.

A bus bombing often requires a fairly intelligent bomber. It is his decision where amongst the passengers to sit on a bus, how to blend in with the crowd, and when during the ride to set off his explosives. Forty years ago a popular theory was that bomb would be set off remotely or by a timer in case the carrier "chickened out." This is no longer the reality.

In busy urban situations, the passengers can range from local residents to tourists from abroad. Intercity routes with multiple stops can carry an even wider variety of passengers. This plays a role in DVI. In virtually every bus bombing, there is increased pressure to close the incident even at the expense of standard response procedures including DVI and return the area to normalcy.

In most bus bombings, the local fire department is in charge of site security regarding possible flammability of spilt fuel. Their dousing of the area to prevent conflagration obviously over-rides all DVI considerations for site preservation.

Bus bombers (bombers in general) do not act alone. They are not "lone wolves." They typically are buttressed by a support network that choses the bus line, prepares the explosive, and transports the bomber. The identification of the bomber' body can be extremely important in furthering the investigation to locate the rest of the cell, thus there are occasions in which this identification is given priority.

There are, of course, causes of explosions other than bombings. These range from industrial accidents to faulty gas lines. Many of the DVI aspects are similar (Galante *et al.*).

Chemical Leak

There is no one "catch all" to deal with chemical leaks. Exposure to chemicals can be from a manufacturing process at a factory or even from cargo on an airplane that has crashed.

There are numerous types of chemicals, and each can constitute a different hazard. Dangerous substances pose various health and safety hazards. There are chemicals that are toxic, explosive, flammable, self-reactive, oxidizing, or corrosive. Contamination can be by inhalation, absorption through skin, or ingestion, sometimes with extremely serious effects. It is incumbent on responders to identify any potential chemical hazards before entering a site. For DVI responders, if there is a chemical hazard, it should be clarified if bodies of deceased persons might contain and exude dangerous materials. This is particularly but not exclusively true when performing autopsies (Edkins). The same is obviously true in chemical warfare attacks.

Fire

Burns are categorized as 1 through 5 degrees, describing their penetration into the body. This is a medical definition only partially applicable to DVI.

First-degree burns are superficial, affecting only the outer layer (epidermis) of the skin. The definition was written in terms of treating patients. For dealing with deceased victims for recognition purposes, importance is where the burns are on the body. If the burns are on the face, there are significant questions regarding the validity of personal recognition, even as a supplement to other methods. When burning penetrates further into the body (higher degree numbers), changes intensify, and personal recognition becomes even more questionable.

Fingerprints of a burnt victim can also present a challenge. If there is burning on the fingers, strengthening the hand with an injection can sometimes aid in obtaining fingerprints, but as the degree of burning increases, the possibility of fingerprints decreases. At a certain stage, it becomes impossible.

In a totally burnt victim, retrieving DNA can also be a problem. Such retrieval is not always feasible. In cases of extreme fire, only hard tissues (bones and teeth) may remain for DNA analysis. DNA extracted from these bones and teeth may be highly degraded, making amplification of genetic markers difficult or even impossible. Another problem is that heavily burnt bones are very prone to contamination with external DNA. In extreme burning, DNA is not always possible (Schwark).

It should be stressed that DNA taken from a deceased should not be contaminated whatsoever. That caveat applies not only to collection containers but also to less obvious situations such as partial remains of an unknown number of bodies all intermingled. In 9/11, the New York Fire Department doused the scene numerous times with water pumped from the East River—not exactly the cleanest water in town and quite liable to contaminate DNA from exposed sources.

Flooding

There are numerous causes and categories of floods. Direct causes can be break-age of a dam or storms (e.g., typhoons and hurricanes) with heavy rains. For DVI purposes, the most problematic type of flooding is a flood that is sudden or with very short notice, not enabling people to flee (or unfortunately refusing to seek refuge elsewhere, usually due to disbelief or concern for physical prop-erty). Flooding is a classic cause of death in DVI efforts (Jonkman). Setting aside direct cause, the type of flood very much influences any DVI response.

Flash floods move rapidly, often with force and speed. A common problem with these floods is when they occur in areas favored by hikers, they receive no real notice to flee. Search and rescue can be time consuming, and the dead are often washed down stream, sometimes with considerable damage to the body.

Coastal floods strike at a shoreline, often from a storm that is generated at sea. There usually is adequate notice to seek higher ground or flee from the area. A tsunami is classically generated by an earthquake, but it is a coastal flood (wave or waves), often providing little advance warning. It can be highly fatal.

River floods build up slowly. There are usually very few fatalities unless a dam or other protective measures suddenly fail.

Urban floods are caused by failure of a city's drainage system to absorb heavy rain. The lack of natural drainage in an urban area can also contribute to flooding. There is usually significant physical damage but few fatalities. There are, of course, exceptions; however, large numbers of dead requiring disaster deployment are rare.

As can be seen, the geography of flooding can be a consideration in DVI response. In the 1 September 2021 Hurricane Ida made landfall in the Greater New York area, and 11 persons drowned in their basement homes or in their vehicles due to insufficient drainage; the bodies were relatively straight-forward to locate and identify, since they were recovered in places associated with their lifestyle pattern. (In total, some 82 persons died due to Hurricane Ida, 26 of whom perished in Louisiana. A medical examiner deter-mined that 10 were due to heat exhaustion, not a difficult DVI issue.)

Islands and coastal areas mean the victims can be washed far from their original locations; retrieval can be a time-consuming process. The longer a deceased is in water, the faster the body can decompose and be distorted. One initial effect is bloating.

Landslide

Landslide is a very general term. Different professions have various terms and nuances for the phenomenon. In any event, there are several different types of landslides in professional nomenclature (fall, topple, slide, spread, and flow), some with direct implications for DVI (Highland). An alternative word for landslide is avalanche, very often used for snow. Another variation is a mudslide, such as the one that killed at least 96 people in Petrópolis, Brazil on 16 February 2022.

A typical cascade tends to be abrupt with little warning. Large boulders can tumble, jump, and roll until their velocity is slowed by flat ground. A fall can pose building damage and be life-threatening to anything or anyone in its path. Slides can be very fast, but more frequently they are not as rapid. Hence, there is more warning and fewer casualties or fatalities. In short, different landslides generate different dangers.

Landslides can be caused by many factors such as heavy rain, tsunami, volcanic eruption, or earthquake, burying victims in a cascade, flow, or tumble of dirt, vegetation, and/or rubble. This means that landslides often occur simultaneously with other hazards. For example, there have been landslides that have blocked rivers and effected dams (Ataie), causing serious damage. This is yet another example promoting an "all hazards" approach in disaster planning.

The DVI problems encountered in a landslide can be complex, and the exact scenario must be taken into consideration. Many landslides take place on unstable ground or near landfill where less expensive housing is too often built. Defining the "closed population" potentially effected can be cumbersome due to inexact record keeping. An example of a waste landfill landslide occurred in Shenzhen, China, on 20 December 2015, causing the deaths of 69 persons and another 8 persons unaccounted for. A common cause of death is suffocation, but physical damage to the body resulting in critical injury is also frequent.

In an avalanche, the force of tumbling snow can destroy buildings causing fatalities. As snow begins to melt or temperatures rise, water makes the snow heavier, and the increased weight can cause buildings to collapse. An example is the case of the four-story Hotel Rigopiano in the Italian Alps on 18 January 2017, when an avalanche weighing an estimated 120,000 tons struck the hotel at a speed of around 100 km/h. (It is surmised that a partial cause of the avalanche was seismic activity.) Fatalities were 29, survivors 11.

The avalanche posed problems effecting DVI. It took time to first locate the site and then find possible survivors and the dead. Helicopters could not be used because of stormy weather. Roads were blocked by snow. The hotel was buried under at least 13 feet of snow. The command center with ambulance waiting was located 6 miles (10 km) away. After two days, contact was made with six survivors, certainly taking precedence over dealing with the dead. Cold temperatures delayed body decay, but the waiting and uncertainty took its psychological toll on both relatives and responders. Psychologists trained in emergency psychology assisted both families and responders for eight consecutive days. Not to be forgotten, an appropriately quiet venue had to be found for psychological intervention (Pescini).

As can be seen, in many landslides response is slowed by damage to the general area infrastructure (roads, utility lines, etc.).

Trampling

There have been numerous disasters with deaths due to trampling (stampede, crowd crush). On 29–30 April 2021, 45 people died due to trampling at Meron, a religious site near Tsefat (Safed) in northern Israel. In general, most injuries were to the head or internal (Henn). That usually means fewer problems in DVI, provided that *AM* information is available. Even so, there was tremendous family pressure on DVI staff for unreasonably quick identifications.

The immediate cause of a stampede is panic. This can be induced by a factor such as perceived danger (e.g., fire). The situation can be aggravated by weather (a very hot day). Less apparent causes are poor crowd management planning and site architecture. There are sites (e.g., the Kaaba in Mecca, Saudi Arabia, Church of the Sepulcher in Jerusalem, Church of the Nativity in Bethlehem) that have religious significance and cannot easily be redesigned to meet modern safety standards despite repeated crushing disasters. On 24 September 2015, over 2000 pilgrims were crushed to death during the Hajj in Mecca. Primary identification was by DNA, but reports indicate there were problems obtaining proper *AM* samples from abroad.

Command 7

From the very onset of a disaster response, there must be a clear chain of command. It must be evident which organization holds overall responsibility and which person holds ultimate decision-making authority. This also holds true for each and every player. When there is more than one DVI team active in the field, there must be one person in charge to coordinate DVI efforts. In other words, there must be a clear hierarchy at all levels.

During a response it is very likely that personnel will change with shifts and tasks will be added, and by the end of the response closed down. Throughout all of these stages, communications regarding chain of command are critical.

Chain of command authority must take into consideration emergency situations that can arise during response work. If, for example, the fire department identifies an imminent danger and orders immediate evacuation, protocols must delegate authority that overrides the site commander.

This might sound odd, but all disaster sites are not easy to find. A collapsed building or the bombing of a bus on a busy urban thoroughfare pose no particular problem. At the other end of the spectrum an airplane or ship lost at sea can pose major problems to find. Malaysia Airlines Flight 370, a regularly scheduled international passenger flight, disappeared on 8 March 2014. Only in July 2021 was the aircraft reportedly found at sea.

There is middle ground. United Airlines Flight 232 was scheduled to fly from Stapleton Airport in Denver to O'Hare Airport in Chicago, then continuing to Philadelphia. On 19 July 1989, the DC-10 made an emergency crash landing crash-landed at Sioux City, Iowa, after failure of its tail-mounted engine. Of the 296 passengers and crew onboard, 184 people survived. The aircraft broke into pieces upon landing at the airport. It was more than an hour before one group of survivors was found at a far end of the field. Original thoughts were that they were merely onlookers waving to cameras to attract innocent attention.

Theory says to define the area of a disaster and close it off as one would do with a standard crime scene. That is straight-forward with a limited-area building collapse or a bus bombing but not necessarily practical with an earthquake. The disaster area must be closed if at all possible, realizing that after the Loma Prieta earthquake all of San Francisco could not be sealed off.

DOI: 10.4324/9781003345367-9

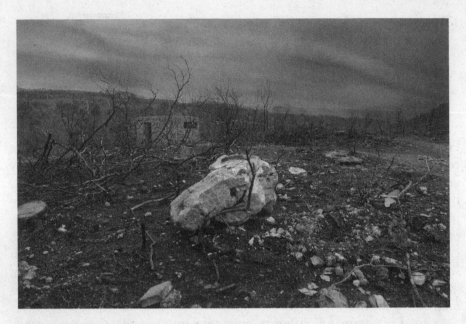

Figure 7.1 A photograph of the devastation from the Carmel fire in Israel, December 2010. In the aftermath, 23 bodies were identified by DNA and 15 bodies were identified by fingerprint.

Source: www.shutterstock.com

In such a case, only selected sites with extensive damage could be cordoned off.

Closing a zone at sea is another matter, not to speak of floating debris and bodies. In the case of Lockerbie, there was no one crash site, and body/debris search was over a vast area.

A raging forest fire is an example of a mobile site that cannot be cordoned off with tape barriers or even metal gates (Figure 7.1).

Rendering a disaster site safe for responders must be handled with protective personal equipment but also when considering the site itself. For example, no personal equipment will protect a responder from building collapse—not in the initial stages of emergency medical treatment, not in later DVI activities. No gloves, disposable gowns, or medical inoculations will protect workers will protect responders from falling concrete. Some dangers also only develop or become apparent in the course of a response.

Safety issues at a site can range from asbestos and silica particles in the air to excessive heat and inadequate ventilation. Not only bombs explode. There is a long list of other chemicals and household items that are flammable. Search of a site for clear hazards is no an activity limited to initial stages.

Safety monitoring should continue throughout the response. It can be prudent to scan responders for health issues after completion of a shift.

Body extrication is not only a function of manpower and equipment. There is a tendency to jump to the quick conclusion that bringing in more teams—in-country or from abroad—will expedite matters. Sometimes that is the case, but in many instances there simply is not sufficient available space to bring in more teams and equipment. This was very much true in the AMIA bombing (Buenos Aires, 18 July 1994), where narrow streets precluded bringing in additional heavy vehicles. In many disasters, extrication is a time-taking operation. It can be likened to a game of Pick-Up Sticks (similar to Mikado), removing a top piece while not disturbing what is below. The basic difference from the game is that by unintentionally disturbing a layer, the site can become unstable and more dangerous.

An Amtrak train collided with Conrail locomotives near Chase, Maryland on 4 January 1987 leaving the engineer and 15 passengers dead. Although the accident took place in a relatively open area, final extrication of survivors and the dead took 10 hours due to the strong frame of rail cars, overturned carriages, and the sheer length of the train. In all, there had been about 600 aboard at the time of the crash.

Another important impediment to rapid extrication can be weather, as was the case after a building collapse (25 June 2021) in Surfside, Florida, where an approaching hurricane caused a work stoppage.

Extrication is an important step in victim identification. There is a temptation to satisfy with quick visual identifications, but that is a non-definitive investigation lead. It should be kept in mind that often the "witnesses" are psychologically unstable and overwhelmed by the incident. There is virtually no end to mistakes in visual identification. Therefore, at least one (if not two) scientific methods are to be preferred, the implication of which is creating a system of scientific *ante mortem* and *post mortem* files and their comparison.

Citizens who happen to be "on the spot" often just "jump in," trying to help. Their intentions are good, their work is invaluable, but in the end, they are not professionals. In one sense, this is a true "Golden Hour" (Granot) in which the most people can usually be saved. Yet these are ordinary citizens. When professionals arrive on scene, they should debrief those citizens concerning what they have done and record contact information. This includes questions that related to DVI.

Professional response including DVI must be a planned activity coordinated with the site commander who receives input from other sources. When the first DVI team arrives, the priority is coordination, ironically not identification. There must be prioritization of activities. After site security from various dangers, often site documentation (photography) is paramount.

There are issues of deceased victims already removed from the point of death, dividing the site into work areas, and timing the entry of DVI teams as well as how many teams can be fielded simultaneously. This means establishing a safe holding area near the disaster site but at a distance so as not to interfere with other response activities.

Ante Mortem and Post Mortem

8

Identification is not possible without adequate *ante mortem* and *post mortem* information collection. The former is usually a police function; most (but not all) aspects of the latter fall primarily in the jurisdiction of a medical examiner.

For example, in police terms, if an identification (often called reconciliation) is to be made by fingerprint comparison, both *AM* and *PM* prints must be available.

Another basic rule of DVI is to collect that significant data that are found most rapidly and lead to a definitive and positive identification conclusion.

It is a matter of work prioritization. If a victim never saw a dentist, charting teeth will generally not lead to a useful finding. Clearly, it is best to find the most recent data if the records change over time. Fingerprints are an example of a feature that does not change, but dental treatment often does change.

If a corpse has no hands, one might think that it is pointless to search for *AM* fingerprints. The exception, of course, is identifying body parts. Such a situation raises a relevant issue. In many cases, an attempt is made to identify all detached body parts. In such instance, locating *ante mortem* fingerprints does have value.

One must keep perspective in determining the importance of body parts. They should be divided into two categories: (1) essential to life and (2) not essential to life. Identifying a torso, for example, is sufficient to prove death. Identification of a detached hand, though, only proves presence of a person in a disaster. Such a body part does not in itself prove death unless it can be shown that detachment without medical treatment would cause non-survivable loss of blood.

Even identification of a body part not essential to life does indicate that the person in question was somehow present in the disaster.

The collection of *AM* and *PM* information can be done simultaneously, and there is no Golden Rule as to which will be faster or easier. This is very case-dependent. The *AM* collection is based on probable victims. *PM* is primarily collected in the mortuary.

DOI: 10.4324/9781003345367-10

In an efficiently laid out program (stations), it is possible to work on more than one body at a time.

Fingerprint Development

Taking fingerprints from a corpse in good condition is relatively easy, but there can be complications. A natural psychological reaction to crisis is to clench a fist. Thus, releasing the fingers can constitute a challenge. This cadaveric spasm often relaxes after several hours; however, there have been cases in which injecting a muscle relaxant was done. (This should not be confused with clenched fist syndrome sometimes occurring after a serious stroke.)

In cases of burning or bloating of the fingers, a fingerprint expert as opposed to a routine technician should be called in.

Statistics

It is very difficult to pinpoint which methods of identification are most frequently used. The answer is very much time-dependent and incident-specific. Disasters before the era of DNA reflect a different reality. The sinking of a ship cannot be compared to a building collapse. Even one air crash can be very different from another. Swissair crashed at sea, and there was no fire. Air Canada Flight 797 from Dallas/Fort Worth International Airport to Montréal Dorval Airport on 2 June 1983 was diverted to Cincinnati/Northern Kentucky International Airport. The cabin was engulfed in flames, killing 23 passengers.

A great deal depends on what happened in the disaster. Type or severity of injury can be a determining consideration in the identification method. After the crash of TW 800 (17 July 1996), for example, remains of all 230 victims were recovered, and injuries were classified in three categories: (1) Serious: trauma that was instantly fatal (183 of 202); (2) Moderate: trauma undetermined but probably immediately fatal (15 of 202); (3) Minimal: trauma not immediately fatal (4 of 202). (These statistics reflect the situation before all bodies and parts were recovered.) Insufficient remains were found in 28 of the 230 to determine their level of injuries. While some remains showed burn injuries (flash burns), most were relatively superficial and likely non-fatal by themselves. Severity of injury can influence DVI procedures.

Searching for *AM* information starts with the assumption that a particular person is a possible or probable victim of a disaster. The difference between those two terms can be an initial factor in prioritizing investigative particularly when investigators are fewer than the work load.

When a specific person is a possible or probable victim, the search for *AM* information usually starts with the family. Standard forms all ask the usual questions regarding employment, medical history, etc. This should provide information for follow-up, including request for dental and medical records, as well as DNA samples from blood relatives.

Fingerprints provide a touchy issue. Medical and dental files are authoritative, since they are created by a reliable medical professional. There is no reasonable doubt regarding the identity of the patient (perhaps with the theoretical exception of a Hollywood mystery or drama). This is also the case of fingerprints taken as part of an employment application or criminal arrest. Lifting prints from a surface that the person had presumably touched is much more problematic. Did someone else borrow his coffee mug? Did a co-worker sit down at his desk for a moment just to jot something down? Although these possibilities are perhaps improbabilities, they should be taken into consideration.

Modern technology has made some *AM* information searches easier. Biometric passports and identity cards carry verifiable information. In the past, many hospitals discarded patient X-rays after a certain period of time. This was due to storage space and inherent costs. Today digitalization storage is on computer databases (Picture Archive Computer/Communication Systems—PACS) (Shaw). Long-term storage is much less costly. In many cases, a patient is even given a copy for his own retention.

Post mortem data collection is often more straight-forward than *ante mortem*, but the general rule is again, "There is what there is, and that's what there is." A more or less full body makes collecting *post mortem* information for identification easier. Data collection from detached or mingled body parts and burnt cadavers is more difficult. Another rule comes into play. In dealing with body parts, the aim of DVI is to prove death of a person and identify the remains. As noted, proving presence in a disaster (for example, finding a finger of a particular person) does not prove death. The keys are body parts without which life cannot be sustained. Associating various body parts is the job of a pathologist and/or forensic anthropologist. In general terms, the *post mortem* data collection by the police centers around the taking of fingerprints, particularly in more difficult cases.

Today there are many different systems to take fingerprints by scanner. These systems are used primarily as an authentication method to verify identity and permit entry. Many fingerprint experts contend that these systems are not appropriate for *post mortem* fingerprints. This is certainly true with fingers in very difficult condition. There are, however, those who support scanning (Johnson). In any event, those promoting scanning must also set up a capability to take fingerprints manually when scanning is not possible.

In the Mortuary

The mortuary deals with the collection of *PM* information for its subsequent correlation with *AM* information. This includes numerous skills.

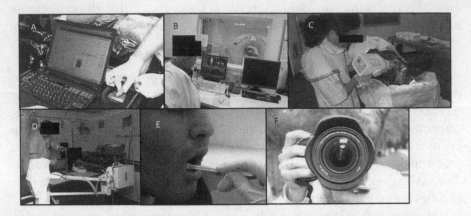

Figure 8.1 PM collection of samples and information from bodies in the collection line at the DVI center. A—fingerprint collection; B—CT of body or body parts for the identification of special marks; C—X-ray of teeth; D—imaging of skeleton; E—swabbing from biological sample used for DNA profile analysis; F—photography of phase and individual body signs.

In routine work, a body is placed on a table, on which workers using various skills handle *post mortem* examination. Each examiner uses the tools that he needs for the specific case. Upon completion of the examination the area is cleaned and readied for the next examination. In a mass disaster requiring the services of numerous experts of various disciplines that approach is not the most efficient. Instead of bringing examination equipment to the body, the body is most often brought to the equipment almost in assembly line fashion. In other words, there are "stations" for examination. As can be seen in Figure 8.1, one typical station would be, for example, for photography. Another would be for fingerprints. The idea is that at each station all of the equipment needed is readily available.

There is no set rule as to the number of stations. That number can be expanded or condensed as circumstances, pace, and workload dictate. Nor is there a rule as to the placement of stations. That very much depends on the contour of the facility being used.

It is important that stations be arranged as much as possible in a sequential order so as to minimize "traffic jams" of gurneys carrying bodies.

Administration

An obvious starting point is registration of the body and setting up an examination file with all necessary forms. At this point, it is decided to which stations a body should be brought. Not all are necessarily needed for every cadaver. A body without hands is clearly not sent for fingerprinting. All bodies, however, are sent for photography.

An administration station is also needed at the end of the sequence of stations to ascertain that all required stations were covered. There the file is put into order prior to being forwarded for reconciliation with *AM* files.

Administration requires forms. As described earlier, the Interpol DVI policy states that these forms be on white colored paper to readily differentiate them from *AM* (yellow) and *PM* (pink) forms and avoid confusion.

The following list of possible stations is alphabetized for convenience and not necessarily prioritized.

Body Description

It is recommended that the first technical station be a general and essentially superficial examination of the body, assessing the degree of injuries and establishing which stations are most appropriate, subject to change during the station-to-station process.

Features to be noted are evidence of prior surgery, blatant cars, tattoos, etc. (There are two types of permanent tattoos. Individual marks are those such as the numbers put on the arms of Nazi concentration inmates. Tattoos used by a group can be the same inscription used by numerous sailors, certain right-wing extremists, or a standard picture bought on a commercial basis. Evaluation must be on a case-by-case basis.)

What is important is that each body be given not only a list of stations to which it should be brought but also a sequence. All bodies must be brought to photography, but few will be brought to forensic anthropology (perhaps with exception of dealing with a mass grave with decaying remains). Sometimes the order of stations is important; sometimes it does not matter; sometimes a station is needed more than once. For example, a body should be photographed as received, not relying on photographs from the field where work is never under ideal conditions. During examinations, there might be need of additional photos to better document a potential identification. Another example is regarding sequence. It often does not matter if fingerprints come before or after odontology.

Forensic Anthropology

Forensic anthropology (Wiersema) is a relatively new field essentially first developed in the 1940s, but now it has a standard place in DVI. Wilton Marion Krogman (1903–1987) is widely credited a being its founder. Krogman was the first anthropologist to stress the forensic use of anthropology to assist in the identification of skeletal remains. Forensic anthropology was used by the U.S. Army to help identify Korean War casualties. This period saw the first official use of anthropologists by federal agencies including the FBI. The primary use of this science in disaster response is with mass graves, skeletal remains, and matching body parts. It is rare that anthropology will have its own independent station during a disaster response. More often anthropologists will be called to assist others. Anthropologists can be key in sorting mingled remains of more than one individual.

DNA

DNA (Deoxyribonucleic acid) has a long history that begins in 1869 with the Swiss researcher, Friedrich Miescher (1844–1895), who was examining the composition of lymphoid cells (white blood cells). He isolated a new molecule that he called "nuclein" (DNA with associated proteins) from the nucleus of a cell. That is usually heralded as the beginning of DNA; however, DNA for identification would come more than a century later. DNA is similar to two strands comprising an almost infinite number of arrangements.

The year 1984–1985 sets the beginning of DNA for forensic identification, when Alec Jeffreys (1950–), working in the Department of Genetics at the University of Leicester, discovered DNA testing to create an individualized marker of a person. Courtroom acceptance of DNA came soon afterwards (Smith) (Figure 8.2).

The U.S. National Institutes of Health has tried to provide a layman's explanation of DNA sequencing. (Forget, "DNA fingerprinting." Sequencing is a more professional term.) A key element in identifying DNA is to establish the order (sequence) of the four chemical building blocks ("bases") constituting a DNA molecule—Adenine (A), Cytosine (C), Guanine (G), Thymine (T). Adenine pairs with thymine, and guanine with cytosine. The order of pairing is almost infinite.

Loci / Sample	FGA	THO1	D19S433	D18S51	D21S11	D8S1179	Amelogenin	D2S1338	D16S539	vWA	D3S1358
Son	21,26	7,7	15,15.2	12,16	30,34.2	13,14	XY	20,21	8,10	17,19	16,17
Mother	20,26	7,9	13,15	12,17	29,34.2	13,14	XX	20,21	8,11	16,17	16,17
Father	21,24	6,7	14,15.2	16,17	30,30	13,13	XY	17,20	10,13	16,19	16,17

Figure 8.2 Identification of DVI based on Short Tandem Repeat (STR) DNA profile of first-degree family members.

Source: The son's STRs fits well with his parents' profiles [For further information, a useful reference is D. Hartman, O. Drummer, C. Eckhoff, J.W. Scheffer, P. Stringer, The contribution of DNA to the disaster victim identification (DVI) effort, Forensic Science International, 205 (1–3), 2011, 52–58].

This reveals the genetic information contained in a particular DNA segment. For example, scientists can use sequence information to determine which stretches of DNA contain genes and which stretches carry regulatory instructions, turning genes on or off. This information is highly individual.

In a certain sense, DNA can be a race against time. A simple way to take a DNA example is a buccal (mouth/inner cheek) swab, but as time passes, the oral cavity of a deceased dries out. Other body fluids are a possibility, but more advanced laboratory methods can become necessary.

There are several current efforts to identify World War I military dead and buried in mass graves. DNA samples are extracted from the exhumed remains of soldiers and compared with a DNA databank from possible descendants.

For the record, DNA has also been extracted from animals. Canine and feline samples have been used to determine combinations of breed.

Fingerprints

Fingerprints have long been used for individuation and identification purposes due to their unique traits (Figures 8.3 and 8.4). Fingerprinting the dead can be very different from fingerprinting the living. Most obvious is that the dead do not "cooperate." They might even show "resistance," as decay and *rigor mortis* set in. Many dying persons clench their hands. Bodies recovered from water also have bloated features including hands. And, there can be severe burning. (Classic mummification as in Ancient Egypt is outside the scope of this book.) These situations require special equipment not usually carried in the routine kit of technician ns; hence it should be available at a Fingerprint Station (Figure 8.5).

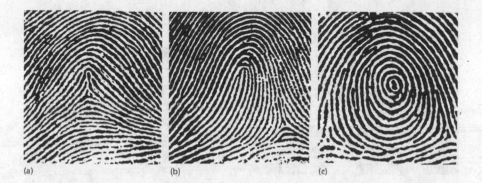

Figure 8.3 Fingerprint patterns: (a) Arch pattern, (b) loop pattern, and (c) whorl pattern.

Source: Howard Harris, Henry Lee, *Introduction to Forensic Science and Criminalistics Second Edition*, Boca Raton, Florida, CRC Press/Taylor & Francis Group, 2019.

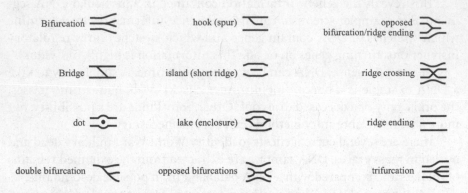

Bifurcation · hook (spur) · opposed bifurcation/ridge ending

Bridge · island (short ridge) · ridge crossing

dot · lake (enclosure) · ridge ending

double bifurcation · opposed bifurcations · trifurcation

Figure 8.4 Each fingerprint presents different topological minutia points: basic and composite ridge characteristics. Comparison can be by an expert or using an automated fingerprint comparison computed system (AFIS).

Source: Howard Harris, Henry Lee, *Introduction to Forensic Science and Criminalistics Second Edition*, Boca Raton, Florida, CRC Press/Taylor & Francis Group, 2019.

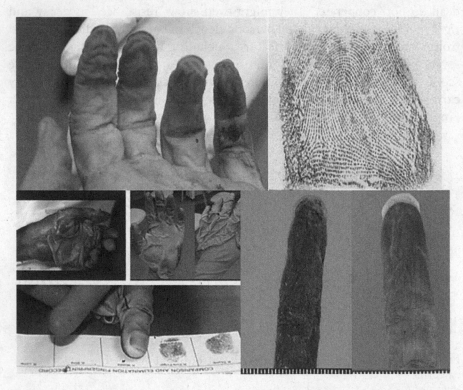

Figure 8.5 Collection of fingerprints from bodies of different conditions.

When fingers are straight or bent/clenched and can be straightened, a hard surface is needed to prevent unintentional movement by the technician as a print is taken. Usually, the inked finger is pressed against a small chit of paper placed on the hard surface. There are companies that sell these inexpensive "kits." To improvise, merely cut short strips of paper, and insert them into a spoon. Labeling, of course, is critical. The ink or powder used is best chosen by the fingerprint technician.

Foot and palm prints are also unique to individuals. Palm prints are sometimes a realistic possibility as a basis of identification (Figure 8.6). Clear prints from the bottom of the foot, however, are often difficult to retrieve.

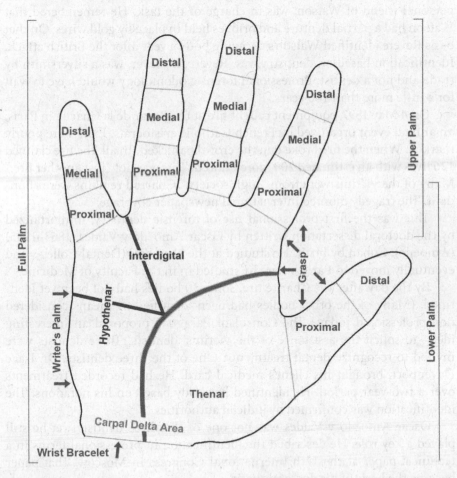

Figure 8.6 The anatomy of the palm: finger and palm segment positions. The palm surface is divided into three zones—interdigital, hypothenar, and thenar—and is compared using the minutia points.

Source: FBI, *A Practical Guide for Palm Print* Capture (Washington, DC: U.S. Department of Justice, 2019).

Odontology

There are numerous historical references to identification by teeth, even dating back to Roman times. One much later example relates to Paul Revere (1735–1818) of Revolutionary War fame.

Dr. Joseph Warren (1741–1745) was a physician and also commander of the Massachusetts militia, killed on 17 June 1775 following the second attack on in the battle on Breed's Hill. The British buried his body in a mass grave. After the battle, the family requested a proper burial for Dr. Warren, given his militia and social status.

Recover the body from the mass grave, but which body? Paul Revere, a personal friend of Watson, was in charge of the task. He remembered that Watson had a partial denture and bridges held in place by gold wires. On that basis Revere identified Watson's decaying body a year after the British attack. Identification based on dentistry, yes. Revere, however, was a silversmith by trade and not a dentist. Professional forensic odontology would have to wait for a little more than 100 years.

On 4 May 1897, equipment caught fire at the Bazar de la Charité in Paris, an annual event organized by French Catholic aristocrats. Exits were poorly marked. When the fire broke out, the crowd panicked. In all, the fire claimed 126 lives with an estimated 200 more injured. This was not "just another fire." Many of the victims were from "high society." Charred remains were abundant. The tragedy merited international newspaper coverage.

This was the first professional use of forensic dentistry, immortalized by the doctoral dissertation written by Oscar Amoëdo y Valdes (1863–1945) (Amoëdo), Cuban by birth. He studied at the New York Dental College, and eventually moved to Paris, where he studied in in the Faculty of Medicine.

By the day after the Charité fire, some 30 bodies had not been yet identified. (Many of the other bodies had been identified by means considered non-professional today.) The Consul of Paraguay proposed an interesting idea—to solicit the assistance of the victims' dentists. Three dentists were invited to recognize dental treatments. One of the three dentists, Dr. Isaac Davenport, brought his client's medical card. He had recorded treatments over a two-year period. He identified her body based on his notations. The identification was confirmed by judicial authorities.

Oscar Amoëdo y Valdes was not one of the three dentists, yet he still played a key role. He described the identification in professional terms in a technical paper at the 12th International Congress in Moscow. That paper became the basis of his doctoral thesis.

In 1899, Amoëdo defended his dissertation, L'art dentaire en médecine légale (Dental Art in Legal Medicine). The reviewers' decision was clear, "This is not a thesis but a treatise on odontology. He filled in all the great gaps which remained in the field *of* forensic identification." The dissertation was published as a book. Amoëdo, the "Father of Forensic Odontology," continued to publish. Forensic Odontology was now a recognized method of identification (Balachander) (Riaud).

At a dental station treatment in the mouth should be charted and sometimes photographed by X-ray or other method. All dentists should be instructed to use the same charting method, of which there are several.

One new examination method is post-mortem computed tomography (PMCT) (Brough) that has been increasingly adopted for dental examination. Its three-dimensional (3D) capability and non-destructive approach offer several advantages over conventional X-rays. As such its potential use within forensic odontology for disaster victim identification (DVI) is under study (Nguyen).

Pathology

Pathology is not always needed for identification. If there are both fingerprint and odontology matches, there is no *identification* reason for pathology, although there might be legal requirements to establish the exact cause of death, usually when the disaster came about by criminal action or negligence (determination outside the scope of this book).

The preferred methods of pathological examination are non-intrusive, thus leaving a body intact. This is because there are both religious and cultural objections to autopsies in certain quarters.

The entire issue of autopsies can be both of an emotional and medical concern. Postmortem computed tomography (CT) is often touted as an alternative and non-invasive procedure. The first practical CT scanner was invented by Sir Godfrey Hounsfield of the EMI Central Research Laboratories in Hayes, United Kingdom by using X-rays, and the first patient brain-scan was performed on 1 October 1971.

CTs, however, have limitations as well as benefits. Research has shown that CTs can show information not seen in autopsies, but the opposite is also true. Autopsies can reveal information not seen in CTs (Leth). A recommended procedure is to use CT before an autopsy (Zheng). From a DVI perspective, if a CT reveals sufficient information for identification, then there is no need for an intrusive autopsy from a DVI perspective.

Photography

Over the years, photography has changed dramatically. Gone are the days of film and wet development. This has also changed the role and function of a photography station.

There are two types of photography at an identification station. X-ray is meant to view features of a body that cannot be seen with the naked eye. Breaks in bones that are revealed by X-ray, for example, can be a definite help in identification. For this purpose, a photography station with appropriate protective safeguards is needed.

Another use of photography is to leave a visual record of findings. Most of this work is done at a photography station. There are, however, instances in which different sections will make a specific request for photography. Rather than wheeling a body, it can be easier to bring the camera to the body. For this reason, a mobile capability should be maintained.

As an incident unfolds any photography possible can help. In a forensic facility, only professional camera capturing details and with excellent focus should be used. One never knows what questions may arise long after a body is identified and buried. These photographs are absolutely different from post-mortem photographs commissioned by a family or used by them to remember a deceased person (Silverthorne).

Property

There are several stages in the handling of property. At the property station in the examination process, all clothing removed from the body and all property on the victim and in his pockets should be deposited into bags, labeled, and secured. The temptation to identify a victim based solely on property must be resisted. Items can be an excellent investigative tool, but nothing more. Preplanning should also determine a protocol for property collection and specify the unit to which items should be remanded.

A personal document or laundry mark found inside the shirt or trousers can lead to an erroneous conclusion. How many people give away clothing that no longer fits? One of the author's daughters wears a ring inherited from a grandmother whose initials are still inscribed on it.

A driver's license in a wallet or a passport in a pocket may match the victim. Excellent. Tempting. But verify it with an examination of the body. Leave no doubt. There are enough cases of people traveling on bogus documents or presumed identities.

Property includes watches, rings, wallets, and even chits of paper found in the pockets. Everything must be placed into secure bags that cannot be opened without signs of tampering and then labeled. At a later stage this property will be matched, if possible, with items strewn at the disaster site.

Although some sources recommend otherwise, experience shows that clothing should not be laundered unless there is a medical decision of possible contamination either from disease or from body fluid leakage. Likewise, personal effects such as jewelry and watches should not be cleaned except for identification reasons or medical considerations. Final disposition of these items is the decision of surviving next-of-kin. In Jewish law, for example, there are situations in which a victim's unlaundered clothing is buried with the victim.

For the purpose of DVI, personal property is significant. In an air crash, for example, personal property includes carry-on and checked baggage as well as items worn and carried in pockets or a handbag. Airplane parts and commercial shipments are sometimes of interest to other responders. In the crash of Thai Airway Flight 311 on approach to Kathmandu on 31 July 1992, most property recovered was from a commercial shipment of clothing, not really of importance, since its condition did not make it saleable. It is essential that all personal property be collected, registered, examined, and eventually returned to grieving family. Often that property is cherished as memorabilia of the deceased.

Cleaning of property after victim identification should be the decision of the family, unless such cleaning is for health, evidentiary, or association purposes. The entire issue of property highlights the need for cooperation amongst various players.

X-Ray (Roentgen)

Many major discoveries were made by accident, not by intention, and X-rays are just one example. Wilhelm Roentgen, Professor of Physics in Bavaria, discovered X-rays in 1895 totally be accident while investigating if cathode rays could penetrate glass. He covered a cathode tube with heavy black paper; then something unexpected happened. An incandescent green light was seen on a nearby fluorescent screen. Further investigation showed that the light penetrated many objects but not solids. Soon it became apparent that these rays revealed bones in the human body. The finding spread quickly as a medical method to observe such features as broken bones and later applications for dental treatment.

In some countries, this procedure is named after its inventor, Roentgen. He, himself, called them "X-rays." X for "unknown."

Accolades poured in, and Roentgen was awarded the first Nobel Prize in physics in 1901. Realization of a critical side-effect, however, was missing. Only decades later were side effects of X-rays identified. Today the use of X-rays is wide-spread. Discs have replaced film for recording images, but there are no shortcuts to protective measures. In DVI terms, the search for *AM* X-rays can be extremely important. *PM*, however, is different. There is no worry about exposure of a cadaver to X-rays; however, the technician must take care to protect himself from the radiation. In practical terms, this means that X-rays may be taken in a facility with appropriate protective conditions.

Temporary Mortuary Facilities

There are times when the number of fatalities in a disaster grossly exceeds the capabilities of a local facility, both in terms of manpower and space. Adding experts is usually handled through professional contacts or bureaucratic channels. Space is a totally different question. What can a forensic institute do when its workload of several bodies a month suddenly expands to dozens in a matter of days? There are generally two options.

The crash of Air Inter is an example in which bodies were stored in two temporary refrigerated tents near the disaster site and then transferred in small groups to the standard facility in Strasbourg. A slight variation is bringing tents or containers to the forensic facility. (There is a psychological rejection for truck containers. If it becomes known that they had been used to store bodies, there is a reluctance to use them afterwards for food despite extensive cleaning.)

Swissair, Pan Am, and a military helicopter crash in Israel show an alternative approach—setting up a temporary forensic facility. There are problems in this approach. The facility chosen in Lockerbie for the Pan AM response was a large school; drainage in one of the "stations" proved to be problematic. In the helicopter response, some bodies had to be brought to the standard forensic facility for use of equipment that could not be moved.

Swissair showed that specific examinations (in this case DNA) could be sent to various laboratories in this case throughout Canada; however, bodies should not be distributed amongst examination sites, so an overall perspective of the disaster can be achieved.

Identification and Cooperation 9

Police cooperation is very often a critical part of disaster response and DVI. There is no guarantee that all victims of a disaster are local to the site. In today's mobile society, people move around for tourism, family visits, business, or other pursuits. This is true not only of air crashes, but it also describes other seemingly local events.

The case of the 25 June 2021 building collapse in Surfside, Florida is a good example. Although the building was essentially a condominium residence, not all victims were residents. Several were visiting family and came from elsewhere. Even the permanent apartment owners raised interesting issues. Some lived elsewhere for part of the year; their *ante mortem* data was not always to be found in Florida. The same can be said for the many immigrants from abroad, primarily Latin America, countries in which *ante mortem* records could be found (not to speak of close family who could provide descriptions in addition to records).

Given this situation, it is obvious that cooperation between police departments even far from each other is critical. A partial solution is to remember that every local disaster response plan must take into consideration that victim identification must include cooperation with other departments, whether by asking for information or answering requests from others.

The overriding rule is that identification must be made by a positive comparison of *ante mortem* and *post mortem* data of significant importance. A major question is what constitutes significant importance. This is very much a variable determination based on several factors including cultural norms and practices. For example, naval piercing is common in some societies but virtually unknown (or even forbidden) in others. Again, cooperation comes into play, as there is often more than one method needed (or preferred) for identification.

In a disaster involving a closed population, any feature applicable to only one person can be considered significant. For example, age can be significant if a closed population includes all adults and one child, and a deceased is clearly a minor. In an open population or with a large group of people, significance is not so clear cut. Culture can be a determinant in assessing importance or significance. In DVI terms, examples can be clothing worn,

DOI: 10.4324/9781003345367-11

nose piercing, or male circumcision. There are, however, certain physical features that are universally held to be unique to only one person, hence significant. The most common methods of identification are DNA, Odontology, and Fingerprints.

DNA

Today many people jump to the conclusion that DNA solves all identification questions. There can be no doubt. DNA sequencing is a potent tool, but it has its limitations. Amongst other considerations, properly functioning equipment and qualified personnel are essential.

"Quick and easy" are mottos of today's life. This may be applied to cooking in the kitchen, but not necessarily to forensic results. There are various DNA kits on the market. The first kits not to be used for forensic purposes are commercial DNA genealogy packages made to assist in building family trees. These should absolutely not be used for forensic purposes including DVI. Accuracy is often a poor 60%.

Professional DNA field kits can be useful for rapid investigative results, but they should never be considered conclusive. There is no substitute for full analysis in a properly equipped laboratory.

DNA results can be wrong! Primary reasons are contaminated example receptacles, faulty equipment, and human error.

The costs of DNA Testing for a crime lab are hard to determine. There are cost savings per examination by scaling up the number of samples, but there is also cost of running a lab and personnel costs together with supplies such as reagents and special chemicals. All of this and more goes into computing sample costs. Normally you need only two specimens, one unknown and the other a known exemplar. If they match, case closed. If not, additional known specimens must be added until a match is found. For an unidentified child, one or both parents are asked for DNA specimens. One parent is sufficient but both parents would be ideal. Commercial specimen testing can range from $500-$2000 depending on whether the example is simple (blood or saliva) vs. decomposed skeletal remains.

Not everyone is willing to provide a DNA example even after a disaster. In this author's experience, one person refused to give a DNA example from fear it would open Pandora's Box and reveal which children were truly related to whom.

Nor are DNA examples always available. There was also a case of a lonely senior immigrant from abroad with no known relatives. No *AM* DNA samples were to be had. (His final identification was essentially circumstantial based upon his declared travel plans and property found at the disaster site.)

As in all DVI cases, there are the standard components of *ante mortem* and *post mortem*. In one case, a DNA example was available only from his wife—invalid since a wife is not a blood relative. She was, however, able to certify which toothbrush was his, and that no one else used it. The toothbrush was taken from his home and served as the source of an *ante mortem* example. More common, however, are saliva examples taken from blood relative(s) (parents/children, siblings, aunts/uncles/nephews/nieces, etc.). The closer the relationship, the better.

In every case, *post mortem* examples are controlled by "What there is, is what there is." In dealing with a relatively intact deceased, DNA is straight-forward, often necessitating only a one-to-one comparison with a specific missing person. Charring and burning can present difficulties. Detached body parts usually require a search of the DNA database created in the specific disaster (a "closed population" created from DNA examples of blood relatives).

Professional DNA sampling kits with supplies for saliva sampling and record keeping should always be kept in adequate supply and be readily available.

Odontology

There is a classic question if any dentist is qualified to establish identification by dentistry or if a forensic odonatologist is required. ("Odontology" is derived from Greek; "Dentistry" is derived from Latin.) Without denigrating the dentist, one must take into account cases in which significant dental work was performed between the filling out of *AM* and *PM* records. A forensic expert is to be preferred. As Dr. Howard Glazer explains:

> A forensic odonatologist is more than just a dentist since he has been trained to see the dentition and surrounding structures in a more specific way. One could compare them to being a "dental detective" who looks at the oral environment for clues relative not only to identification, but sometimes relative to cause of death.
>
> (Glazer)

Dental morphology can be used as a suggestive tool to determine the race of a victim; however, it should be used with caution.

Advantages of odontology are that, like fingerprints, it can be relatively inexpensive, rapid, and definitive.

Fingerprints

Fingerprints are unique to every individual, and they do not change over time as skin regenerates itself. Even identical twins have different prints. They are also unique to every finger. In other words, no two fingers have the same print. In very basic terms, there are three very general categories of fingerprints: loops, whorls, and arches. (There are several types of whorls, making it the most common category.) Differentiating them is based on fine details. An experienced examiner can usually determine which finger has left a print.

Over time there have been numerous fingerprint classification systems (Cole). One of the most commonly used was the Henry system, developed in the early 20th century primarily by Sir Edward Richard Henry (1850–1931), for many years the Commissioner of the Metropolitan (London) Police.

Computerization has made the Henry system obsolete. Today's standard is the Automated Fingerprint Identification System (AFIS), the first version of which was released in 1986. At first numerous manufacturers tried to market their products. Since then, however, the number of manufacturers has dwindled. Here it must be remembered that the computer searches and suggests. It does not "compare and decide." AFIS only "suggests." It certainly does not replace the qualified fingerprint expert.

Not to be forgotten is another fingerprint skill—the ability to take *PM* prints from bodies in difficult conditions. This is not within the expertise of the average fingerprint technician, who is trained to lift latent prints from a crime scene or take prints from suspects or other live persons.

For the record, toe, foot, and palm prints are also unique, but they are rarely used for identification. Some hospitals take footprints from babies. They are taken by nurses, not at all by professionals, and they are often blurred and unreadable.

Other Medical

In addition to the aforementioned techniques, there are others that are equally definitive. Many medical treatments can be significant for both positive identification and negative exclusion. In the former case, comparison of AM/*PM* invasive surgical procedures can be decisive in establishing identification. In the latter case, if the deceased had his tonsils removed, but they were intact in the victim's body, this is obvious exclusion.

Features such as broken bones (with X-rays of exact breakage) and physical malformations are also important.

These and other medical determinations are within the competence of forensic pathologists.

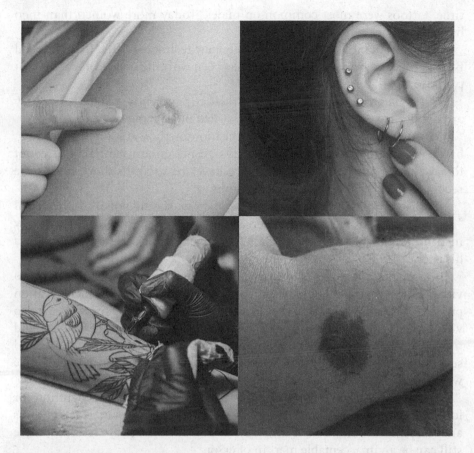

Figure 9.1 Typical individual marks on bodies: pathologic external marks, scars, pigmentation, tattoos, etc.

Source: www.shutterstock.com

Miscellaneous

Numerous questions arise concerning significance. There can be external marks such as scars, jewelry pinned to the ear and/or nose, or tattoos (Figure 9.1).

Is a permanent tattoo significant? (Rub on and wash off have little value.) Yes, and no. Some are, and some are not. Many sailors on ships often have the same tattoo, whereas concentration camp prisoners during the Holocaust were given very unique numbers. Gangs often have the same tattoo on their members. If a person was known to have had a tattoo, but none was found on that place on the body, this can be sufficient for exclusion. There are methods for tattoo removal; however, usually permanent light scars remain. At one time, tattoos were most common on males. Today more women than men have at least one tattoo.

Identification by tattoo is a relatively new technology. The U.S. National Bureau of Standards and Technology has been working on a protocol for that purpose.

Paste-on or rub-on tattoos have little if any evidentiary value, since they are not permanent and can be readily washed off, leaving no trace.

An important factor in any identification method is a forensic finding, based on a feature on the physical body and not circumstantial. This is not to say that circumstantial evidence can never be used. In short, it must be recognized for what it is and its limitations.

Disaster responders, whether police of other, should not allow the visual "identification" of victims—neither at the disaster site nor at a pathology institute. This is perhaps appropriate for a small traffic accident but not for a disaster.

Personal recognition is a very sensitive subject. Some relatives want to view a body, when at all possible, as part of what they feel is the identification process. It can also be part of the closure process. Viewing, however, can also yield serious consequences. In one case in Israel, a close relative sent a friend to view a body after a bus bombing and confirm identification. That friend sent to view the body suffered a heart attack. As a lesson learnt, an ambulance was stationed as standard procedure when viewing bodies after a disaster.

A basic question revolves around the validity of visual recognition for identification. The problem is twofold—the psychological state of the witness and the physical condition of the body. Even if both issues are resolved, there still can be an unacceptable margin of error.

Viewing the body of a friend or relative is by no means a pleasant experience. In evaluating a person's testimony, his psychological condition must be taken into account. Even if the witness appears to be stable psychologically, trauma is still possible. Some witnesses want to close the matter quickly and do not look carefully, even though it is *they* who requested the viewing, perhaps for closure, perhaps as a culturally acceptable norm, perhaps just to say goodbye.

A preferred procedure for visual identification (even though this is not recommended as definitive, but can be complementary) is to sit with the witness and ask what the person expects to see. Are there scars? Beauty marks (melanocytic nevus)? Where on the body? The next stage is to bring the witness to view the body and show the examiner the identifying features that he/she had described verbally. No words of caution are sufficient. This procedure is aimed at the psychological condition of the witness. Visual identification in mass disasters should be used only as supportive evidence (if at all) or to service survivor needs. It has been prone to mistakes.

Another problem with visual identification is with the condition of the body. Not all remains are appropriate for viewing by friends or family. Not only is recognition impossible. It can also intensify traumatic reactions. The decision to allow viewing is essentially that of a medical examiner.

Viewing a body found in water poses unique problems. Even time in the water before body recovery can influence decomposition and changes.

Looking at a picture of a deceased even for preliminary identification also raises problems. People are three dimensional, and photographs are not. We see people from different angles, but a photograph is taken from one perspective. These are just two reasons why one cannot rely on photography.

There is an idea that photographs can be of preliminary value in selecting the body that an identification witness will be invited to view. A pitfall is that the witness may psychologically decide on the identification already in the stage of the photograph.

Photography

The role of photography in DVI is not a simple subject. Some photographs, essentially used by medical professionals, pose little problem. These include a wide variety of X-rays, from dental scans to features in other parts of the body (e.g., pictures of fractures or mal-formations). The basic question arises in general photography of the body.

It is recommended to photograph bodies at the disaster site as soon as possible, since all bodies change and start to decay as time passes, particular in hot weather or after they are recovered from water. Computational comparison of AM/PM face photos may be considered (Figure 9.2).

After one disaster in which it was decided not to show a damaged body to a father, he was shown a picture of a unique mark on the victim's leg. One might attribute his rejection of the evidence to denial, but his stated reason was that the color was not quite right in the picture. After seeing the actual mark on the body, he broke down crying and said, "Of course!"

Investigations

Investigations are integrally tied to DVI. Identification is based on an *AM/PM* positive comparison. DVI technicians can collect *PM* findings from the scene for later use by a potentially wide scope of experts. Those specialists can suggest the most useful *AM* information needed for comparison, but it is the task of police investigators to locate that data. In a routine case, a medical examiner might well pick up the phone and request medical records (in accordance with local privacy laws); however, with the overwhelming workload of

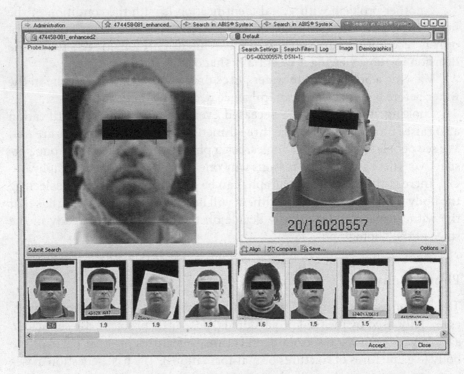

Figure 9.2 Computational face comparison/recognition in photo album.

a disaster, that role invariably falls on police investigators. The search for *AM* fingerprints also reverts to DVI and its fingerprint technicians, particularly when it means lifting latent prints from a victim's home.

There are, of course, other roles as well for investigations. Investigators should be stationed in area hospitals to record the arrival of injured persons from the disaster site. When hospital staff determines death, notification should be made to the disaster information center for further processing in addition to standard procedures for the issuance of a birth certificate (if the deceased has been identified).

All persons involved in a disaster must be accounted for, whether they be healthy, injured, or deceased. Although DVI relates to deceased persons, general investigation is broader, particularly if a crime or criminal malfeasance is in question.

Data Corroboration (Reconciliation)

10

The matching of significant *ante mortem* and *post mortem* information is called data corroboration or reconciliation. The best way to do this is to use complementary *AM* and *PM* forms with numbers that are matched, such as the INTERPOL forms.

Quality control can play a determining role in reconciliation. As part of the identification decision-making process all data should be verified as belonging to the victim under consideration. The physical quality of data should be verified. For example, fingerprints should be sufficiently clear and not blurred. Items compared must be of sufficient importance.

It is best that a second opinion on identification be rendered to avoid possible error. In a disaster response, even key decision-makers can be under unusual stress and can make mistakes. If, for example, identification is based on forensic odontology, a second dentist should check the findings. Fingerprint comparison is another example. Mistakes can be made due to pressure or overwork (Grosse).

An important consideration is if an identification is based only a body part, it should be determined that the part be essential to survival. A written record of the decision-making process should be made in case later question arise.

Next-of-kin should be notified not only of the identification but also of its basis to remove any doubts they might have regarding identification. In the United States, the Aviation Disaster Family Assistance Act states that the air carrier is primarily responsible for family notification and all aspects of victim and family logistical support in air disasters; however, the Act is ambiguous and leaves leeway for other arrangements. The cause of death must be in terms that that the bereaved will understand. Clear terminology can be quite difficult in cases of fragmentary, decomposed, or burnt bodies, but specifically in these situations the bereaved are most in need of convincing evidence. This can be a critical stage in acceptance of the identification by the bereaved.

It is not the task of a DVI technician to make a notification of death. Even in cases of anticipation, the notification can cause extreme reactions. This is best handled by persons trained for the task. Only afterwards can a DVI

DOI: 10.4324/9781003345367-12

representative be called upon to explain the situation and basis of identification (Cohen).

The crash of Eurocopter AS365N2 Dauphin helicopter in Malaysia on 4 April 2015 raises a procedural question. At what point should families be notified of an identification? Most of the six identifications were based on highly convincing secondary evidence, and at that point families were notified. Only later were the identifications verified by DNA comparisons.

Many people want to view a body. This can be "to say goodbye" and/or to theoretically verify the identification. When the physical condition of a body allows such, viewing can be a helpful step toward closure, even though it has very little true value in identification.

After one bad experience in Israel (heart attack of a close friend viewing a body), it is standard practice to have paramedics and an ambulance stationed outside the building in which the bodies of disaster victims are viewed.

For the record, there have been cases in which the wrong body to be sent for repatriation was presented for viewing due to a mix-up in paperwork. One of those cases was in Lockerbie.

Computerization

Computerization of *AM* and *PM* data is best done when the number of fatalities exceeds the efficacy of manual systems in both input and search time. Once again computerization means cooperation between players. Although DVI might select a program to be used, it is most frequent that computer experts tend to the technical aspects of running the program.

Manual input of data should always be checked for typing accuracy. Computer searches can be one-to-one, *AM* driven, and *PM* driven.

After a computer data base is organized, a one-to-one comparison can be made if a specific body is thought to be that of a specific person. The search is made to confirm a particular presumption.

AM and *PM* searches are made when there is substantive information, and one wants to know if it matches any information in the data base. This can be either to suggest a match or as an indication of a possible identification that needs more investigative work.

As in other computer searches in many fields, a "match" is a mathematical probability and suggests, not makes, an identification. Only an expert can certify an identification. There are several commercial companies that offer computerized data systems. Some are restricted to a specific discipline such as odontology. A popular general product is KMD PlassData, headquartered in Denmark, which is integrated with INTERPOL forms and procedures.

It should be remembered that computerization of DVI is not necessarily desirable in all situations. If it is professionally decided to computerize a database, only a well-tested and reliable program should be used. Again, pre-incident preparation is necessary.

Confirming Identification

A common question in victim identification is how much information is required to establish an identity. Is a positive fingerprint match sufficient as sole evidence? Is a second method also to be preferred? Without any doubt every effort must be made to avoid errors or conclusions based on suggestive but not firm evidence. Whenever possible, a confirming method based on sound scientific methodology should be used to remove all doubt about an identification. Although this may slow the pace of work, it is certainly more preferable than trying to undo an error. It is simplistic to say that confirmation must be by a second primary method (odontology, fingerprints, and DNA). This might be theoretically desirable, but sometimes it is neither practical nor possible. It is better to say that the second method must be "decisive." One should shy away from mathematical models computing projection of probability (such as Bayes Theorem) when dealing with combinations of weak data.

Body Release

Bodies cannot be released until they have been identified, cause of death determined, and a legal death certificate issued (Speers). Part of general disaster planning should be a procedure to issue official death certificates for fatalities without bureaucratic delay. If the jurisdiction issues death certificates in a local language not commonly understood elsewhere, official certificates or translations should also be provided to avoid later complications.

Cause of death is outside the realm of DVI; however, its importance cannot be overlooked, since it may later be a necessary element in legal or insurance proceedings as well as any safety-related investigations. Specific cause of death is the responsibility of pathologists.

There have been mistakes in body release, sending the wrong body to a family. One such mistake was caught at the last minute following the Lockerbie crash, when friends of a deceased acting as agents of the widow inspected and saw they were being given a casket with the wrong body. A guideline is that body release can be a stressful task in disaster response, often handled by people with no prior experience. It is by no means akin to a clerical task of logging out material.

In typical Jewish legal proceedings to prove a person's death and release a spouse to remarry, cause of death is a standard question in addition to identification of the deceased. This is asked so that an orderly and complete file can be built supporting DVI findings.

In many cases, there is no DVI reason to show a family what remains of a body. There is also good reason for them to even know how much remains or in what condition. After one plane crash involving intense fire, only charred flecks of skin remained on the bones retrieved. Before body release, the coffin was filled with dirt to approximate the weight of the deceased to obscure the body's condition from the family.

Beyond Identification 11

Standard DVI guides produced by international organizations or even individuals tend to be a reflection of Western culture. There are also many publications that have stressed scientific principles without taking into consideration human factors such as social values, religious tenets, and personal closure by the bereaved.

DVI is not a textbook procedure. There are religious requirements of bereaved families. One might take the "professional" attitude that police and pathology methods are definitive and beyond reproach. Anything more is the problem of the family. True, but not true. This contradicts another principle—that the police must serve the public. It is not unreasonable to contend that the police must attend to mourners' needs to any reasonable extent. There are, however, many unreasonable requests.

Western culture dictates that identification can be as rapidly as possible, but within a professional framework. There are endless newspaper accounts of bereaved families complaining about slow body recovery and identification. The complaints can be reasonable, emotional, irrational or a combination of all of the above. There can be, however, underlying issues.

In Chinese culture, visiting the disaster site and returning by a circuitous route to ward off an evil spirit take precedence over rapid identification (in many cases even over providing *ante mortem* information). Some interpretations of Islamic Law stress rapid burial, even at the expense of technical and scientific identification. A respected Islamic cleric in Israel contended after a bus crash that if one victim is Moslem, all victims should be treated as Moslem, understandably a request that could not be accepted. Traditional Jewish Law has very specific requirements for body identification, often precluding visual identification. Other religious representatives have declared that they accept all police decisions about identification, not examining the nature of the identification and the quality of the service providers.

There are clergy with different types of professional training. It should be noted that although clergy can play a very effective role in disaster response (Massey), their training rarely includes expertise in the requirements even in their own religion for disaster victim identification, and not all members are appropriate for disaster response tasks. Those trained for congregational functions are most suitable for disaster response, since they most often have

DOI: 10.4324/9781003345367-13

experience dealing with congregants in crisis (Feldbush). A problematic tactic in one disaster was to use the clergy as a "psychological protection" eliminating direct police (DVI)-bereaved interaction.

Although faith oriented, clergy are not immune from burnout and adverse psychological reactions (Jackson-Jordan). There are NGOs that deal with the religious needs of families in times of disaster; their services can have implications for DVI by calming the relatives to supply accurate *AM* information. It is insufficient to call upon NGO volunteers to deal with bereaved families just because they are willing. They must be trained for the task.

NGOs and clergy often deal with the families of missing persons; those families are invariably the source of critical *ante mortem* information. In many cases, those outside sources deal with the psychological needs of the families. Only when those family members are relatively calm and not hysterical can the police ask that DVI questions be posed and get responsible answers.

Closure

Disasters are not just large traffic accidents. Their implications are very different. In a typical traffic accident, body recovery is relatively rapid. The victims' identities in a traffic accident are usually known relatively quickly. In a mass disaster, retrieving bodies can take days, weeks, or months . . . if at all. In a mass disaster, matching missing persons' reports to possible victims can be a prolonged endeavor.

The death of a close relative or friend is always traumatic. In a disaster, there is no warning. It is not like a person whose health was declining. Even then it takes time to psychologically adjust. After a disaster, the uncertainty involved in waiting for an identification has its psychological toll. Maybe he wasn't there? Maybe this? Maybe that? When death is the realistic or final conclusion, the process of closure begins.

There has been significant discussion regarding the meaning of closure. Suffice it to say that in the context of DVI, closure is coming to terms without doubt and reservation that the person involved is dead (Kübler-Ross 1969). Linguists have analyzed the euphemisms of death (no longer with us, met his Creator, passed on, etc.) to soften impact (Rawlings *et al.* 2017) and facilitate closure. From the limited point of view of DVI, unequivocal confrontation with the fact of death, without any uncertainty, is needed. Otherwise, people can reject forensic findings and retain unrealistic (even the most fanciful) illusions that the person involved might still be alive (Wayland 2015).

Some people can reach closure without outside assistance. There are others, however, for whom closure is a hard-to-achieve goal and require professional intervention.

Sometimes the problems of closure are compounded by financial loss associated with a disaster (Tsuchiya *et al.* 2017). One example is destruction of a home in which the deceased lived. Collecting remaining possessions and deciding what to keep can complicate coming to terms with the overall situation. Sometimes closure is made difficult by reassigning daily chores that the deceased used to perform or cleaning out personal effects. In the author's experience, one widow broke down when she instinctively started to buy cigarettes for her then-deceased husband.

Victim identification obviously has legal implications. Death certificates enable next-of-kin to close bank accounts, settle debts, apply for insurance benefits, etc. Not to be overlooked, however, is that the settling of legal matters is a step in the process of closure.

From a wider perspective, closure is more complex than merely the recognition of death. The family of one fireman killed in the 9/11 disaster postponed a funeral ceremony for 15 years, hoping to find his remains (Revesz 2016). This is a classic example of lack of closure. Although the family was convinced of the relative's death, the preoccupation with finding his remains prevented a total return to routine. Searching for remains became a preoccupation.

In many cases, such as airline crashes at sea or military confrontations (Defense 2018), not all bodies are recovered, even though there can be sufficient reason to establish death. Even though evidence can be clear, such cases pose problems of closure.

> Families may feel unable to fully grieve and reach closure in situations when there is no positive confirmation of the death, when the physical body has not been recovered or if the body is available but the family is unable to view it.
>
> (Dyer and Thompson 2010)

Sometimes what would objectively be considered proof of identification is insufficient for the bereaved and precludes closure. After one terrorist attack, pathologists were reticent to show a damaged body to a bereaved family. Instead, they showed a picture of a unique tattoo on a specific place on the victim's body. The identification was rejected, since the color of the tattoo was not quite "right." The family was experiencing "denial." Acceptance and the beginning of closure came only after the color scale was adjusted.

Although the bereaved family is primary, friends can also need closure, since they can feel the loss of the deceased. The same is true for co-workers (APA 2011) and even school children when a classmate passes away.

A family will never achieve full closure (Boss and Carnes 2012) until supporting documentation is sufficient to satisfy what Joseph Scanlon called "other players" in dealing with death, such as insurance companies. A key issue can be determination of benefits and liability in indirect deaths stemming from disaster. Per the Centers for Disease Control & Prevention (2017), this can be particularly controversial in instances such as heart attack or unhealthy post-disaster conditions. Closure often awaits resolution of insurance decisions.

After a disaster in which two persons are killed (simultaneous death), and they are joint owners of a property or one is the beneficiary of the other, there can be complicated rights of inheritance. Again, inheritance issues can preclude normative closure.

In very bureaucratic terms, one might say that professionally based identification is the task of the medical examiner, and psychological closure is the responsibility of a mental health worker. The two tasks cannot be separated. There are times when police DVI personnel are called upon to assist in explaining an identification to assist in closure.

They are many people for whom closure means knowing exactly what happened. It is not only the cause of a fire or building collapse. After one air crash, a widow was concerned if her late husband was conscious during decent to the ground after the aircraft had been ripped apart by a bomb. This was an important element in her search for closure. Criminal prosecution of the perpetrators was of continuous concern. The compensation payment was not so much a financial issue as symbolic retribution.

Closure is also not a one-time experience. As time passes, doubts can be experienced. Longing for the deceased can engender thoughts of "maybe . . ." with kinds of fantasies. One of the purposes of periodic memorial services, mourning rituals, monuments/tombstones, and visits to a grave is to reinforce closure and strengthen the ability to cope with the death of a close relation.

Sometimes memorials have a negative effect and are a point of controversy. In one air crash, a group of 35 students from Syracuse University returning from study abroad were killed, and the school erected a Place or Remembrance in their memory. A graduate of the same university was killed on the same flight, but he was not part of the group. He was not included in a memorial service nor did his name appear on the monument, causing misunderstandings and ill feelings in his family.

Closure is also not final. One report (Snyder 2017) details the travails of a family after a grave was desecrated and the grave stone removed. How did it happen? Endless efforts were expended to regain closure. There was no doubt about death and identification, but a Pandora's Box of questions reemerged, and memories of the deceased began to dominate thinking.

One might contend that family closure is a psychological issue not connected to police identification. The process of closure sometimes begins with denial, taking the form of rejection of an identification or outright non-cooperation.

In one case in Israel, a wife tried to contend that she was "unavailable" to provide *ante mortem* information. Her reaction must be understood. It was obvious that she could not confront the fact that her husband had been killed in an air crash, even though she knew quite well that he was scheduled to be on the flight in question.

More typical problems of closure are post-identification. In a case handled by the Israel Police, a mother was "too busy" to receive details (that she later totally rejected), explaining why her son's body had been positively identified after a mass drug-related killing. Perhaps this is an extreme example, but it raises the question of the role of identification. It is fair to say that members of the identification team should sit with families to explain an identification if the family has any doubts. Psychological challenges in coming to life-style adjustment are best left to trained psychologists and social workers.

When There Is No Body

Unfortunately, not every cadaver is recovered in every disaster. This can be because of factors such as topography, intense fire, or death at sea. In these cases, "identification" means unequivocal proof that the person thought to be involved was definitely on the airplane, boat, or other and could not possibly have survived.

A classic example is the sinking of the Titanic on 14–15 April 1912. There is ample testimony as to some of the missing and never recovered who were definitely aboard the ship. An eight member orchestra reportedly kept playing as the ship was sinking. Only three of their bodies were found and identified. It is plausible to assume that long-term survival in –2°C (28°F) water and intensive rescue searches is not realistic. Even so, the missing Roger Marie Bricoux, a cellist with French Citizenship aboard the Titanic, was charged a year later with desertion from the French Army after he failed to report. Only in 2000 was he officially declared dead.

In perspective, despite extensive studies, there is no definitive number of passengers who perished on the Titanic. Most estimates set the number at *about* or *in excess* of 1,500. Discrepancies emanate from duplication in the passenger list, crossed out entries, and primarily inexact recording of third-class passengers (between 700 and 1,000 according to different estimates).

A modern example is the Thai Airways Flight 311 that crashed in the Himalayan Mountains on approach to Kathmandu, Nepal. All 99 passengers and 14 crew were killed, but body retrieval was extremely difficult given the terrain.

Almost all passengers aboard the flight and their remains were never found. A professional estimate concluded that it was impossible to survive the impact of the crash, and even if so, it was not reasonable to survive in the mountainous terrain. That was step one. Proof of presumptive death also required interviews in Bangkok's Don Mueang International Airport, the point of flight departure. These inquiries clarified processing procedures that showed that the two Israelis did definitely board the ill-fated flight and did not de-board before take-off, a theoretical possibility. There is also an unusual DVI aspect. Identification teams organized to work. Experts were brought in from abroad, but psychological frustration set in. There were virtually no bodies to be examined.

More than 20 years after the attacks on the World Trade Center on 9/11, some 40% of the bodies of those declared dead still were not identified. The deaths were established based on testimony and presumption, leaving some bereaved families with difficult decisions and severe problems of closure.

Although we talk of DVI as identifying the dead, "victim" can include when there is no death. After the 7 April 2022 terrorist attack in Tel Aviv, Ichilov Hospital needed assistance in identifying two wounded persons who were unconscious.

Social Worker, Psychologist, Psychiatrist, and DVI

There are numerous professionals who assist disaster victims and their families. The primary ask of a social worker is to assist victims and their families with psychological support and guidance through the bureaucratic maze that follows every disaster. The bureaucratic maze can be a complicated, frustrating, and challenging process. This can take the form of maximizing on local response resources, insurance claims, death benefits, and of particular importance in DVI, suggesting psychological treatment for bereaved persons in need of such. A social worker can provide consoling support but not medical treatment.

Not every social worker is trained to deal with the bereaved. There are numerous paths of training such adolescent behavior, old-age problems, family relationships, financial need, etc. The "right" social worker must be chosen. Even then social workers should be watched for any of *their* adverse reactions when dealing with bereaved families.

A clinical psychologist can be a key responder in various disaster response roles. When a social identifies a problem that is beyond her field of expertise a logical next step is to call in a psychologist. Referring a person to a psychologist is a crude way of saying, "You have a problem. You need help." The procedure should introduce the psychologist to the bereaved (Cohen).

Another role of a psychologist is on site to observe the behavior of responders. DVI responders are particularly vulnerable to problematic reactions such as bewilderment, confusion, and distancing. After all, the policemen are not accustomed to mass disaster sites that can be much more overwhelming psychologically that a murder scene or fatal traffic accident. Even as a DVI technician leaves a disaster site, the psychologist should strike up a conversation to monitor reactions. Another conversation should be held a few days later. In the case of problems, sometimes raised by the responder, the psychologist can recommend or commence treatment (Cohen).

A psychologist cannot necessarily solve all problems. Referral to a psychiatrist is an option. Only he can prescribe medical treatment. This is not an exaggerated scenario. There are cases in which psychiatrists have even recommended hospitalization for extreme reactions to disaster. Those reactions can and have resulted in heart attack and suicide (Cohen).

Dealing with Acts of War

A superficial analysis presumes that the military builds an identification file for every soldier sent into battle. The thesis is generally true in modern societies, and the military identifies its fallen soldiers, but there often are loopholes in file regulations. Often the procedures do not take into account administrative staff working at logistic and support locations thought to be "safe," and civilian contractors performing functions far from front lines.

Death in battle can differ very unpleasantly from passing away from illness in a hospital bed. All too often advanced forensic methods or even difficult fingerprint comparisons are available only in police forensic laboratories and not in the military infrastructure.

Experience has shown that even use of military identification files can be problematic, since staff members (soldiers) can calculate height incorrectly, weight can change, and fingerprints can be blurry. Police requests for military identification files are possible in many countries (though often regulated), as law enforcement needs information to verify DVI decisions.

Civilian deaths as a result of military action can be difficult to prevent even with the existence of precision weaponry. Often these civilian fatalities cannot be treated as routine police cases, since the specific location of the bodies can be under threat of continued enemy fire. Even in cases of more or less intact bodies, scene documentation is performed by the military, not the police. This is all the more so in complex body extrication scenarios as a result of wartime bombing.

Determining the status of a victim—military or civilian—can be a politically charged issue as in the case of the 2021 Israel-Gaza fighting. Research has shown the fallacy of unreliable and politicized identifications of "victims." Some of the "civilian" victims were belligerents in civilian attire. Others were killed by friendly misfire, more conveniently attributed to enemy action.

Thus, the identification of these casualties is far from routine and should not necessarily taken at face value.

Dealing with Terrorism

The aim of a terrorist is to cause fear and disrupt daily life as much as possible. In an urban bus bombing or a bombing on a main highway, typical examples, clogging streets with major traffic jams is part and parcel of intentions. The longer the disruption and inconvenience, the better from the perspective of the perpetrator(s) (and there is usually more than one to work through scouting, site selection, bomb preparation, etc.). If the terrorist is killed, rapid and definite identification is critical from an intelligence perspective to reach the other members of his cell.

Police response to terrorism is complex. On the one hand it must simultaneously block traffic and cordon off the incident site, while at the same time clear a path for emergency vehicles to both arrive and depart, also providing alternate routes for the flow of routine traffic and unblock the inevitable traffic jam. There are, of course, vehicles that must be parked, such as police. In incidents in both Kansas City, Missouri (Hyatt Regency skywalk collapse, 17 July 1981) and Cove Neck, Long Island, New York (crash of Avianca Flight 52, 25 January 1990), police cars parked quickly by hurried first response had to be towed away.

"Scoop and run" (quick evacuation of the injured by ambulance) is not always practical.

Often, an area is needed to preform triage—establishing priorities and determining the necessity for medical treatment as well as choice of the most appropriate receiving hospital. Time is needed, space is needed, and traffic personnel must reroute vehicles. Alternative streets might be available for cars, but not necessarily for busses and trucks.

The political response aim is straight-forward (and often dictated via the police)—return the area to normal as soon as possible. The implications for identification are profound. Scene documentation and body removal can be quicker than identification technicians would like. Scene cleanup, particularly on main streets and intersections, is often hastened. Identification information collection is often subservient to broader political considerations and priorities.

Without question, the saving of lives takes precedence over every other consideration. That means that in the bedlam of response doctors and paramedics disturb the scene, moving and removing victims, strictly against procedure in a typical murder scene with no one alive. In addition, there are other complications. Often fire workers are inspecting and dousing the area to prevent further conflagration as bomb experts inspect the scene for additional explosives.

The public should not be forgotten. In case after case, members of the public are, in essence, the first responders before professionals arrive. This includes passersby as well as those lightly or not at all injured. Their work is not to be criticized. Again, their goal is to save lives, not to preserve evidence.

There is a caveat that should be remembered. After terrorist incidents, DVI can take on major importance if there is to be prosecution of the perpetrators. In many jurisdictions, it is insufficient to present charges of murder by merely counting bodies. The prosecution must provide the names of specific victims, i.e., DVI conclusions. In more usual instances, insurance companies can request proof of death in addition to a standard death certificate before a benefit is paid.

Psychology cannot be ignored. There is a definite negative psychological effect of a disaster, particularly a terrorist act, on the ordinary citizen. The longer the incident continues, the psychological effect only intensifies. This is another incentive to wrap up a response as quickly as possible, even at the expense of additional DVI documentation.

Part of closing an incident is cleaning the site. No matter the method of cleaning (washing into a drain/sewer or careful cleaning by volunteers), this action means that all on site DVI actions are ceased.

As has been mentioned, human mains have the potential to carry disease. This should be taken into consideration when cleaning both indoor and outdoor surfaces exposed in particular to body fluids (a common phenomenon after a disaster and violent death). Equipment such as brooms, bushes, and floor "mops" should be made of non-porous material such as silicone, then washed thoroughly with soap or detergent after use. Best is professional equipment in which bristles remain separate and return quickly to their straight position, so that infectious agents do not remain after disinfecting.

Bereaved

Body identification very often requires the assistance of close family relatives, whether it is in filling out victim description forms, providing *ante mortem* medical records, giving DNA examples, or visually identifying the deceased. A classic reaction is for out-of-town family to rush to the city of the disaster, often given complimentary passage by an airline following an air crash. In many cases, this means leaving *ante mortem* records at home.

In most instances, these family members are cooperative as would be expected, even though their functioning may be limited by the confusion and emotions typical of crises situations. Cooperation, however, is not always the case. After one air crash, a widow reacted, "We were getting divorced. Speak to my lawyer." Another widow asked, "I am his second wife. Do you have to tell his first wife?" In another case, a widow complained about supplying *ante mortem* data, "Can't this wait until tomorrow?"

Negative reactions and lack of cooperation even extend to body repatriation even after identification. To quote one widow, "I hate him. I don't want him dead or alive." Sometimes an overt reaction of apparent cooperation hides a quite different reaction. In one case, investigation showed that a disaster victim had been on his way to notify his wife that he was divorcing her after a rocky marriage. The wife carried on as though she never had problems with her now deceased spouse, thus hiding perceived stigma from a divorce (Levinson).

Burial, Exhumation, and Cremation

In most jurisdictions, burial or cremation are family decisions and totally outside the realm of victim identification. There have been cases in which the previously identified dead have been exhumed after questions arose. Sometimes the concern is identification. Exhumation has also been ordered as part of a criminal investigation. This option, clearly, does not exist after cremation. In many countries, cremation is a big business with an accompanying selection of urns in different materials, sizes, off-the-shelf design, and painting on special order.

It is generally concluded that DNA disappears after the intense heat associated with cremation. Extracting DNA from teeth or bones is not possible in a standard cremation, since these body parts are pulverized and subjected to extreme heat (Harbeck *et al.*).

In essence, burial is usually not a DVI decision; however, there might be an exception. In times of war or health emergency, there is a concern of temporary burial (single plots and not mass graves). In this case, bodies are buried rapidly with the intention of exhumation (and formal DVI to verify initial identification under field conditions) after fighting has ceased.

Mass Graves

There are numerous reasons why people are or have to be buried in mass graves. It is a fallacy to surmise that this practice is restricted to past history. It happens even today. In many cases, there are attempts to identify the dead, albeit not necessarily to be classified as *disaster* victim identification.

One motive for creating a mass grave is rapid burial for health reasons in times of wide-spread sickness and plague, thus limiting the possibility of contamination. An obvious reason is war dead, primarily enemy soldiers and civilian fatalities; however, there are cases of mass burial of one's own troops. Another reason is to hide a crime of mass murder, for example the Holocaust and the Rwandan genocide of 1994 (Haglud *et al.*).

Management of mass grave exhumations is very different from usual mass casualty situations. There is often a political dimension to the effort, and there is no pressure to save lives. In cases of proclaimed genocide, political thoughts must be excluded in favor of pure professionalism. The team is also different from standard DVI. It includes archaeologists, anthropologists, and pathologists as well as security personnel, logisticians, heavy equipment operators, photographers, surveyors, dentists, mortuary managers, etc. (Skinner).

There are cases in which an anthropologist is needed to sort remains (often bones) and reconstruct individual bodies. This is necessary before many identification efforts are undertaken. Another task of an anthropologist is to separate non-human bones also recovered (O'Donnell).

Other DVI Responders 12

There are varied reasons why a country will send its DVI team abroad in addition to humanistic motivations and pure altruism.

As Israel was first setting up its DVI capability, representatives were sent to an earthquake in Armenia (7 December 1988) and the crash of Pan AM in Lockerbie to learn how a disaster is handled. This learning process included attending a seminar hosted by the FBI in Quantico, Virginia, and surveying the response to the crash of Air Inter near Strasbourg, France based upon a research grant. DVI presence at the disasters was for learning and not rendering assistance.

Another type of learning is learning by doing. It is not unknown (but not prominently publicized) that a country will dispatch a DVI team abroad for members to gain experience for response to a future potential disaster at home. This also provides an opportunity to test equipment and work protocols.

Often a country is motivated by a sense of responsibility for its citizens thought to be victims of a particular disaster. In such a case, a DVI team is dispatched to aid in the collection of *post mortem* data and reconciliation with *ante mortem* data collected at home or provided by the host country. Needless to say, all possible assistance should be rendered to the host country without restriction by citizenship unless so requested.

Individual politicians have been known to lobby for the dispatch abroad of a DVI team based on personal interests such as the possible involvement of a friend or family member. This can be considered as the usual pressure of a politician, but it should not be decisive in a professional DVI decision.

A repatriation team can also be tasked with returning a body to the home country; however, a DVI team has much broader responsibility. After proper advance co-ordination (usually involving the Foreign Offices of the two countries involved) (Zadok), the team often joins with the local DVI effort.

When multiple countries dispatch DVI teams to the same disaster such as a wide-spread earthquake, each team is generally assigned a specific area. Most common is for all teams to work using the same protocols, most often those of Interpol. There must also be an agreed upon usage of terminology to avoid misunderstandings.

There are, of course, teams that are sent for purely political reasons, usually as a friendly gesture to the host country. Although the basic motive

DOI: 10.4324/9781003345367-14

might be calculated and pragmatic, it should not have any real influence on DVI (or other) operations.

Professional expertise (e.g., dentistry and fingerprints) is one basis of selecting the team to be sent. Language capability is also a key factor in dispatching a DVI team abroad. It is not necessary that all members of the team speak the language of the destination country, since their work is professional/technical. Nevertheless, it is best to have a translator working each shift, rather than relying on host country translation. Sometimes translation can be through a commonly understood third language such as English or French. Mistranslations can lead to misunderstandings.

Terrorist attacks in particular are politically charged events that can evoke local sensitivities to foreign DVI teams. After the AMIA bombing, this writer was asked by the local police why the Israelis were collecting information (*AM* data) on Argentinian citizens. He was also summoned to the Supreme Court to explain the DVI process and related activities including the collection of *AM* data.

Outside Aid and Contractors

Not all DVI services are available in every police force or other governmental source. Sometimes a country will ask for foreign governmental assistance, for example through Interpol or directly from another government. Alternatively, there are countries that volunteer their assistance. There are also private companies that offer identification services.

A pioneer in commercial identification service is Kenyon Emergency Services that began in 1906, when a London and South Western Railway train jumped its tracks and crashed in Salisbury, England. Brothers Herbert and Harold Kenyon of JH Kenyon Limited deployed assistance from London to work with the Coroner and Chief Constable to prepare and repatriate the deceased. Today Kenyon International, sold by the family in 1996, is a well-known service provider, ranging from pre-incident training to disaster response (Jensen).

There is, however, a potential ethical problem of supplying personal data to a private concern in conjunction with disaster response (Knoppers *et al.*). Legal concerns tend to evolve around chain of evidence, particularly in cases in which criminal intent (e.g., bombings) or building code violations are involved. A recommended procedure is that data and files be transferred from police in one jurisdiction directly to police in another jurisdiction and not directly to a private company representing the second police force. The receiving police thereby hold responsibility. That way there is a clear path for security and privacy concerns.

Another ethical question revolves around a private company publicizing details of their disaster response as an advertising tool to promote future business. Not publicizing specifics can also leave the false impression that a company had played an exaggerated role well beyond their real contribution.

NGOs and the Private Sector

An NGO by definition is a non-governmental organization. These organizations have both benefits and drawbacks. NGOs can more easily render assistance in countries with which there are strained or tense diplomatic relations, thus avoiding direct confrontation between governments. This also extends to in-country neighborhoods where official responders can suffer from cultural clashes with local residents. NGOs assisting citizens need to be neither invited nor approved by an official government agency in democratic countries. They often can merely offer their services in functions not provided by governments. It is often sufficient for outside NGOs to co-ordinate arrival with a local organization. In the cases of the Surfside, Florida building collapse and the Tree of Life Congregation (Pittsburgh, Pennsylvania; 27 October 2018) terrorist attack, United Hatzalah from Israel was invited by the local Jewish Federation (Maisel).

An added advantage of an NGO is that they have more flexibility in their operations, since they are not usually hampered by numerous rules and regulations that typify government agencies (e.g., length of working shifts). In any case, however, they should never overlook the main goal for which they were deployed.

A major factor that can detract from NGO functioning is lack of reliable funding as government agencies do have, hence reliance on fundraising. This means that, after an incident, many NGOs need to publicize their roles for fundraising purposes.

NGOs have various motivations for joining a disaster response. Most common is a genuine desire to render help. This is best done when the NGO's activity is integrated into pre-incident planning. Simple examples are ambulance services and food support. There are NGOs that tend to care for bereaved families, travel of relatives, arranging mourning rites, etc. These functions are not directly related to DVI, but they can assist the general process. The smoother the general response is, the better chance DVI will encounter fewer problems.

When care for bereaved families is done with proper coordination, this means that the responders in question are able to relate to families and take an active part in obtaining *PM* information. In Surfside, Spanish-speaking NGO responders helped interrogations and provided translation services.

Not every circumstance can be anticipated. Sometimes unforeseen needs arise calling for an unplanned invitation for an NGO or other organization to assist. This is very different from groups that show up "to be part of the action," as an ego trip searching for publicity, or lacking proper tools such as training or insurance. In one incident in the United States, an uninvited out-of-area DVI team showed up to render unwanted assistance to official government forces. They were sent home but managed to stage a "photo op" to fundraise amongst the unwitting.

There have been instances of over-response, when unneeded forces come before the extent of the disaster is manifest. This is rarely main DVI teams, since they are not amongst the first responders and arrive after life-saving efforts and clarification of the situation.

There is, unfortunately, a negative side to using NGOs and other volunteers. When a government official breaks discipline, punitive measures can be taken. That is not so with NGOs. At worst they can be reprimanded and sent home. In more than one instance, an NGO leaked sensitive information to the media, such as DVI identifications before next-of-kin were notified (Tsaroom 2022).

It should be noted that there are volunteers not at all connected to an NGO. This ranges from private citizens providing food and drink to experts in a profession whose services might be needed (Whittaker *et al.*)

Ambulances

Different jurisdictions arrange ambulance services according to local protocol. In the United States, it is most common for ambulances to be dispatched through calls to 911, the emergency call number standard. Once a disaster is declared, ambulances are routinely dispatched to the scene. The general rule is that these "official" ambulances take patients to the nearest available hospital, taking into consideration emergency room space and medical needs. Even when the ambulances are private, they fall into an official category when dispatched through 911.

Private ambulances appearing on their own operate very differently. They are not price regulated, and they can take a patient to the hospital of his (or the driver's) choice on an unregulated fee basis.

Whether an "official" or a private ambulance is used, best practice is to report the destination of each person transported, so that accurate victim locations can be recorded.

There are patients who cannot be resuscitated or otherwise pass away in ambulances heading to hospital. In many jurisdictions, ambulance paramedics are not authorized to determine death, since they are not licensed physicians. Official determination of death is certified at the destination hospital.

Police investigators should be stationed at all plausible hospital destinations to record arrivals. This record is important in keeping track of victims and later in DVI.

Food and Drink

At all disaster scenes, basic personal needs must be addressed. Drinking is clear—hot in cold winter months, cold in the summer heat. Planning might want to limit many sweeteners and caffeine particularly in coffee and carbonated sodas, since these can be linked to causing increased anxiety.

Lockerbie is a prime example of a prolonged operation in which the Red Cross provided without charge 24/7 food for responders with choices of what to eat.

When meals are provided, they must be culturally appropriate for the population and be in consultation with a dietician to avoid or at least minimalize foods that can spike anxiety and depression, common reactions to disasters (DVI workers not being exempt from these reactions). Primary culprits that can increase anxiety and/or depression are fried foods, processed meat, many candies, assorted pastries, refined cereals, and high-fat dairy items. A plant-based diet is recommended (Wien and Sabate).

If a DVI team is flown to a host country with an appreciably different diet, bringing basic food (when possible) is recommended. This is particularly important in disasters that disrupt routine sanitary water and food supply lines.

Post Incident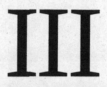

Caring for Responders—
Mental Health

13

DVI workers should be watched for both the onset of psychological issues both during and after a disaster. Not all problems emerge immediately. Problematic reactions to disaster are normal.

Although fatigue is usually considered a physical issue, at a disaster site it can be both physical and psychological. A work day at a disaster site is not necessarily an eight-hour shift. It can be less. One recommendation is 5 to 6 hours including rest periods (Amar). It is the responsibility of a supervisor to determine efficient usage of available manpower to keep teams working around the clock in shifts if necessary (Tsaroom).

Psychological stress was once called battle fatigue, then Anxiety Disorder. Since the 1980s, this phenomenon has coined this Post-Traumatic Stress Disorder (PTSD) based on DSM-III-R (American Psychiatric Association), a key guidebook for psychiatrists.

PTSD is the quite normal but excessive psychological reaction to an unpleasant event. Its manifestation can take numerous forms—such as confusion, nightmares, disorientation, memory problems, fatigue, headaches, pains, anxiety, guilt, denial, emotional outburst, inability to recall an important aspect of the event(s) ("psychogenic amnesia"), and behavioral changes. Sometimes these behavioral symptoms occur while working (and should be spotted by team members or attending psychologist). Sometimes those begin only post-incident. The problem can exist for hours, days, weeks, or even years. Responders should be screened more than once for the necessity of professional psychological intervention. DSM-V has updated aspects of PTSD.

In the experience of the authors, several DVI responders hesitated reporting personal psychological reaction to superiors out of fear that these phenomena might hamper their professional careers. The behavioral reaction is understandable but wrong. All health issues, whether physical or psychological, must be reported and treated. Psychological trauma is absolutely normal, and pre-incident training must describe it as such.

PTSD is not necessarily akin to a bad dream that just goes away—sometimes yes, sometimes no. Again, personal experience, not book-learnt theory, recalls a case in which PTSD led to a fatal heart attack. In another, it was a

DOI: 10.4324/9781003345367-16

strong influence causing marital problems at home. These are hard issues to prove, but that is not a reason to decline or avoid treatment. Here the burden falls in major part on co-workers (team members) who are in the best position to spot problems. Professional psychologists should also be present to look for problems.

Even psychologists sent to deal with families after a disaster can suffer from PTSD. They, too, are not immune. Some psychologists are better suited for research or standard clinical work and not for disaster response (Maisel).

There are numerous approaches to PTSD. For some individuals, it is best to suppress traumatic memories. Airing memories can lead to a variation of personal secondary traumatization. For others, it is more advantageous to speak about what they saw and did. Sometimes airing out the past comes only after years of suppression. (This same reaction can be seen in many Holocaust survivors who refused to talk about their experiences but to talk or write memoirs only after many years had passed.)

A common manifestation of PTSD is general fear. A trip to the grocery might lead to a serious traffic accident. A routine medical examination might uncover a fatal disease. There might be a catastrophic earthquake. One treatment is Cognitive Processing Therapy, developed in the 1980s and used extensively by the U.S. Veterans Administration, typically in 12 weekly sessions either for a group or for an individual. The first four sessions deal with the theory of CPT and trauma. The next three focus on the connection of events to reaction. The final sessions are concerned with safety, trust, power/control, esteem, and intimacy.

PTSD is not only triggered by what one sees. It can also be traced to what one hears—the stories of survivors of a traumatic event.

Caring for Responders—Physical Health

There are many misconceptions regarding health hazards posed by cadavers. The hazards are for the most part to be anticipated but often promoted or exaggerated by the press and emotionally gobbled up by the public. The main threat is after an epidemic, not the type of disaster that poses problems of victim identification. An objective understanding of infection can prevent unnecessary anxiety by both response workers and bereaved families.

Death after air crash, building collapse, or earthquake is most likely caused by physical injury, suffocation, fire, or drowning—not infection. Nevertheless, protective gear should be used by on-site responders, since there are hazards stemming, albeit not common, from diseases such as tuberculosis and HIV carried by the dead even though there is often a limited life to the infection.

Tuberculosis, for example, is rare today and its germ can die within 48 hours of the carrier's death. There is considerable professional debate if precautions should be taken in disaster response. A similar debate concerns the wearing of masks. Yes, or no? In an average case, the mask does more to assuage fear than to actually protect the wearer.

The biggest health hazards when documenting a disaster site are physical contact with a deceased, his feces, or his blood. Gloves, therefore, should be worn. There are numerous types and grades of protective gloves, often latex or nitrile. The gloves should be flexible for work such as taking fingerprints from a deceased, and they should not rip easily. One size does not necessarily fit all. Responders should also be careful not to touch one's face, wipe one's forehead, etc., after contact with the dead.

Another practical danger is stepping on a sharp item. The most obvious problem is contracting tetanus. Hard bottoms on boots are a prudent example of protection, as are heavy gloves when moving metal. Tetanus can also enter the body even from small open cuts, so long sleeve shirts are recommended.

Scaling Down

Scaling up is a *theoretically* simple procedure. As the scope of a disaster and its response challenges become known, modular units can be added in segments as the situation unfolds. That means proper pre-incident planning.

One of the hardest decisions in an incident response is to decide when to scale down and cease activity. Often there is public pressure to keep working at full strength. When does Search & Rescue stop? When will DVI field operations cease or merely phase down? Sorting through all rubble at the World Trade Center took months. Continued presence of DVI teams on site was simply impractical. At what point do you stand down and return to daily activities?

A relatively easy decision on site is to stop people-related activity when all victims and property have been accounted for, but determining that missing persons are not to be found is not as clear, particularly in an open population scenario. There often is a contradiction between public demands and professional incident assessment that also takes into consideration such factors as personnel exhaustion and important routine responsibilities.

It is usually the decision of the head pathologist in an institute of forensic medicine to halt unsuccessful efforts to identify a victim, but that only means that the file is transferred to an appropriate police unit. In such a case, it is clear that police DVI technicians and investigators return to their routine functions.

Debriefing

Short debriefings after a shift can be useful to clarify successful/unsuccessful procedures and to help identify personnel staffing issues. In depth debriefing after the incident must be standard procedure. These debriefings must be held at several levels—DVI, and the various levels of site activity and management. For example, there should be a post incident accounting of DVI/logistics interface, DVI/medical evacuation experiences, etc. These reviews should form a basis for revised working rules.

It is recommended that a psychologist be present at all debriefings particularly involving personnel physically present at the disaster site, so that he can identify any psychological reactions that require follow-up. Sometimes even off-site support personnel victims encounter problems. After one air crash, the policeman managing a chart of identified and not-identified victims suffered from PTSD and retired several months after the incident. He never saw a body. He never met with a bereaved family.

Only the Spokesmen Talk

The media wants news. That is their *raison d'être*. When news is not provided to them, they will use their own resources to find a story. It is the role of spokesmanship to provide news and fill the void.

Media coverage follows a pattern. The initial news photos are heartbreaking and initially usually concentrate on emotional scenes. Very often initial reporting is exaggerated. After all, that is not only a typical response. It is what attracts an audience. The second stage in the media is usually casting blame—delinquencies in enforcement of building standards, delays in on-site equipment supply, and perceived delay in medical team response time. Fortunately, sometimes there are heroes who risk all to save others. Yet there is one story that continues long after the public has lost interest in splashy headlines and heart rendering tales—casting blame.

Do not necessarily blame the media! Often reporters on the scene suffer from the same problematic psychological reactions as other responders, and their initial reporting can be more emotional than factual.

Theory states that only a designated official spokesman releases information to the public. The rationale is clear. In the case of victim identification, next-of-kin should be notified of a death before a public announcement is made. All official announcements are also supposed to be reliable for accuracy, and any pictures released to the press should be screened for "good taste." That is according to the rule book, but in today's world of communications not everyone plays by the rules. Traffic accidents attract much less attention, so premature notification is rare. Disasters, however, present a totally different reality. Sensation and news scoops can often over-ride etiquette.

A major complaint against official spokesmanship is that it is slow, too slow for many media outlets. Information must be verified for accuracy, and notification to bereaved families takes precedence over the public's "need" (or better phrased "want") to know.

When there is a void, it will be filled. When there is no official news, the media will find alternative sources. If there are no other sources, conjecture and rumor take over. This media practice cannot be radically changed easily, if at all. It must be recognized as a working reality. Another working reality is passersby invariably have telephones with photography capability and messaging to multiple addresses simultaneously. Information can be impossible to control as it once was.

Very few media reporters have extensive experience in disaster response and victim identification. Their background is usually general knowledge as an aware citizen and previous disasters (few, if any) on their beat. Another theoretical approach is to periodically brief reporters in case a disaster will occur. This is impractical theory. Almost no one will be interested. Most often the briefings will never generate a story.

There are spokesmen who are well versed in disaster response—for example, those who organizations routinely dealing in responding to disaster, such as the Red Cross and FEMA. In most cases, it is best for a spokesman to have a ready and up-dated list of potential contacts expert in the various aspects of handling disasters, so that reliable background is quickly available. The work of a good spokesman begins long before an issue (any issue—not necessarily related to disasters) arises. He must be prepared if he has to deal with a wide range of subjects.

In many scenarios, the media is viewed almost as a spokesman's adversary. That is unfortunate albeit too often true. When handled properly the media can be an essential element in the constructive delivery of important and accurate information to the public.

During a disaster response, there are numerous organizations that are involved, each one wanting to highlight and publicize its own role (Figure 13.1).

An NGO providing logistical support might want to focus on the many meals they serve. A local municipality is usually interested in focusing on the effectiveness (true or false) of their emergency planning. It is only natural that each group looks after its own interests. There must, however, be overall coordination, so that sensitive information is not released prematurely. That means an overall spokesman to provide guidelines and assist the media in finding appropriate spokesmen. Media representatives like to quote different sources, even if they are saying more or less the same thing.

In terms of victim identification, spokesmanship must be coordinated between the police and the medical examiner. In the most frequent cases, there is a process in media coverage that starts with "what happened," then

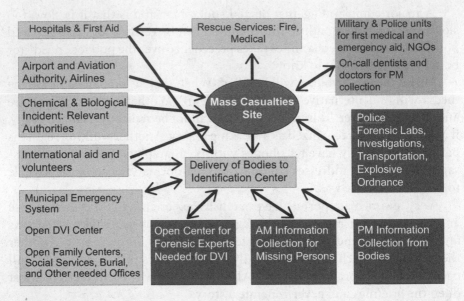

Figure 13.1 Organizations at a DVI Mass Casualty Site. All organizations and agencies should be integrated into one objective.

moves to the missing, extrication efforts, those identified, hours and as normalcy returns criticism politely couched in elective praise. The identification process really does not interest the public other than "fingerprints," "DNA," etc.

In dealing with spokesmanship, one must realize that there is more than one audience, and that must be taken into account in the planning process. One audience is domestic in the country in which the disaster takes place or whose citizens are involved. Not so simple. A terrorist attack in Israel has at least two domestic audiences—Jew and Arab, each viewing the incident differently. There is also an international audience with significantly different interests. One must also take into consideration spokesmanship in different languages.

DVI must be dealt with by a spokesman. Problems in body extrication must be dealt with. Delays in identification must be clarified to the public to create an impression of diligent work and the need to notify families before releasing names to the public. The domestic audience is more interested in the names of victims than international media unless a famous personage is involved.

Spokesmanship should not end with the closing of the incident. One should consider the historical record. Call this public relations. Call this spokesmanship. The appellation is not important, but the historical record *is* important. There must be a clear post-incident presentation of exactly what happened in terms of both statistics and activities. This will serve as a late analysis of the incident by outside scholar and project an image of the responding units. It is important that DVI not be overlooked.

Lockerbie provided an early example of post-incident spokesmanship, in this case probably more accurately dubbed public relations. A film was produced to explain the incident and its response. Image projection was clearly a motivation, rather than recording a full and accurate recording of events— successes *and* failures. This approach of highlighting success and ignoring failure is often reinforced by principles in the response who present papers at professional conferences and submit articles to journals, selectively retelling the event. One could frankly (facetiously) say that for many the disaster becomes the dominant event in their otherwise routine careers.

The engagement of the media with DVI should not end with the last identification. There still is a story, important but of lesser public interest and certainly not sensational. On the anniversary of the tragedy, the media might well look back. With the benefit of retrospect, what lessons were learnt? Were all of the victims, in fact, identified? Were both general and DVI responses adequately funded? The past should provide lessons for the future, and it is the role of the press to inform citizens of issues that should be addressed by government.

Is the era of social media a help or a hindrance in DVI? Does social media violate privacy concerns? In essence, there are no controls regulating social media—not for accuracy, not for good taste. In many ways, social media are uncontrolled and uncontrollable. One cannot lock every transmission and censor every (or any) photograph. It is a situation with which one must simply cope. A partial antidote is for spokesmen to avail themselves of social media to disseminate accurate information and authorized photographs.

Before Closing the Book

DVI is a dynamic field. Proudly we can all say that DVI of today is not DVI of yesterday. Much has been learnt. New and improved methods of identification have been introduced. There is every reason to believe that even the near future will see new methods. Innovations, however, should always undergo sound review before they are adopted or practical use. The ramifications of correct DVI are serious. Identification of a deceased can not only release property and financial or insurance payment. It can also enable a spouse to remarry. Identification methodology must be sound. There can be no mistakes.

No recommendation in this book is absolute, nor is it necessarily applicable in every situation. Each disaster is different. Jerusalem has suffered several bus bombings. There are similarities, but each is different. Police deployment and DVI can be influenced by time of day, alternate traffic routes, and even the width of a street so that sufficient response vehicles and equipment can be brought in. Recommendations are not rules. They are preferred suggestions. Specific response must always be adjusted to the disaster being handled.

In one sense, the book is never really closed. One should not organize a file, discard seemingly extraneous notes, and say, "Done." All notes and seemingly duplicate photographs should be saved. One never knows what questions will arise, or what future lessons may be learnt.

Bibliography

Al-Madharic, A., & Keller, A. Review of disaster definitions. *Prehospital and Disaster Medicine* (1997), 12(1): 17–21.

Amar, S. Interview with Levinson, 20 July 2021 in Maale Adumim, Israel.

American Psychiatric Association. *Diagnostic and Statistical Manual of Mental Disorders: DSM-III-R* (3rd edition, revised). Washington, DC, American Psychiatric Association (1987).

Amoëdo, O. The role of dentist in the identification of the victims of the catastrophe of the "Bazar de la Charité". *Dental Cosmos* (1897), 39: 905–912.

Ataie-Ashtiani, B., & Yavari-Ramshe, S. Numerical simulation of wave generated by landslide incidents in dam reservoirs. *Landslides* (2011), 8(4): 417–432

Balachander, N., Babu, N.A., Jimson, S., Priyadharsini, C., & Masthan, K.M.K. Evolution of forensic odontology: An overview. *Journal of Pharmacy & Bioallied Science* (2015), 7(1): S176–S180.

Black, S (Ed), et al. *Disaster Victim Identification: Experience and Practice*. Boca Raton, CRC Press (2011).

Brough, A.L., Morgan, B., & Rutty, G.N. Postmortem computed tomography (PMCT) and disaster victim identification. *Radiology Medical* (2015), 120: 866–873.

Buck, D.A., Trainor, J., & Aguirre, B.E. A critical evaluation of the incident command system and NIMS. *Journal of Homeland Security and Emergency Management* (2006), 3(3).

Byard, R.W., & Winskog, C. Potential problems arising during international disaster victim identification (DVI) exercises. *Forensic Science, Medicine, and Pathology* (2010), 6: 1–2.

Byrd, J.H. Chapter 9 The victim information center and data collection its evolving role in DVI. In *Disaster Victim Identification in the 21st Century: A US Perspective*, J.A. Williams & V.W. Weedn (eds.), Hoboken, New Jersey, Wiley (2022). https://doi.org/10.1002/9781119652823.ch9

Chaturvedi, A.K., & Sanders, D.C. Aircraft fires, smoke toxicity, and survival. *Aviation Space, and Environmental Medicine* (1996), 67(3): 275–278.

Cohen, M. Interview with Levinson, 10 January 2022 at Ramat Aviv, Tel Aviv, Israel.

Cole, S.A. *Suspect Identities : A History of Fingerprinting and Criminal Identification*. Cambridge, Harvard University Press (2001).

Daniel, V. The social history of disaster victim identification in the United States, 1865 to 1950. *Academic Forensic Pathology* (2020), 10(1): 4–15.

DePaolo, F. *The Role of Forensic Science in Mass Fatality Management*. New York, NYC Office of Chief Medical Examiner (2015).

Dijkhuizen, L.G.M., Gelderman, H.T., & Duijst, W.L.J.M. Review: The safe handling of a corpse (suspected) with COVID-19. *Journal of Forensic and Legal Medicine* (2020), 73.

Dumfries & Galloway Constabulary. www.dumgal.gov.uk/article/15211/Preparing-for-emergencies-in-the-community. Accessed 3 April 2022.

Dzeboev, B.A., Gvishiani, A.D., Agayan, S.M., Belov, I.O., Karapetyan, J.K., Dzeranov, B.V., & Barykina, Y.V. System-analytical method of earthquake-prone areas recognition. *Applied Sciences* (2021), 11: 7972.

Edkins, A., & Murray, V. Management of chemically contaminated bodies. *Journal of the Royal Society of Medicine* (2005), 98(4): 141–145.

Feldbush, M. The role of clergy in responding to disaster events. *Southern Medical Journal* (2007), 100: 942–943.

Fisher, J., & Reed, B. *Disposal of Dead Bodies in Emergency Conditions*. Geneva, WHO (2014).

Fitrasanti, B.I., & Syukriani, Y.F. Social problems in disaster victim identification following the 2006 Pangandaran tsunami. *Legal Medicine* (2009), 11(Suppl. 1): S89–S91.

Forrest, A. Forensic odontology in DVI: Current practice and recent advances. *Forensic Sciences Research* (2019), 4(4): 316–330.

Gabbrielli, M., Gandolfo, C., Anichini, G. Candelori, T., Benvenuti, M., Savellini, G.G., & Cusi, M.G. How long can SARS-CoV-2 persist in human corpses? *International Journal of Infectious Diseases* (2021), 106: 1–2.

Galante, N., Franceschetti, L., Del Sordo, S., Casali, M.B., & Genovese, U. Explosion-related deaths: An overview on forensic evaluation and implications. *Forensic Science, Medicine, and Pathology* (2021), 17: 437–448.

Glazer, H (DDS FAGD FAAFS. Deputy Chief Forensic Odontology Consultant, Office of Chief Medical Examiner, City of New York). Email correspondence with Levinson, 15 November 2021.

Granot, H. *The True Golden Hour: How People Respond in Emergencies*. Toronto, Key Publishing Company (2010).

Grosse, I.C. Fingerprint identification: Potential sources of error and the cause of wrongful convictions. *Journal of Student Science and Technology* (2017), 10: 1.

Haglud, W.D., Connor, M., & Scott, D.D. The archaeology of contemporary mass graves. *Society for Historical Archaeology* (2001), 35(1): 57–69.

Harbeck, M., Schleuder, R., Schneider, J., Wiechmann, I., Schmahl, W.W., & Grupe, G. Research potential and limitations of trace analyses of cremated remains. *Forensic Science International* (2011), 204(1–3): 191–200.

Hartman, D., Drummer, O., Eckhoff, C., Scheffer, J.W., & Stringer, P. The contribution of DNA to the disaster victim identification (DVI) effort. *Forensic Science International* (2011), 205(1–3): 52–58.

Henn, V., & Lignitz, E. Kicking and trampling to death. In M. Tsokos (eds.), Totowa, New Jersey, Humana Press (2004).

Highland, L.M., & Bobrowsky, P. *Landslide Handbook—A Guide to Understanding Landslides*. United States Geological Survey and Geological Survey of Canada (n.d.).

Jackson-Jordan, E.A. Clergy burnout and resilience: A review of the literature. *Journal of Pastoral Care Counseling* (2013), 67(1): 3.

Jensen, R.A. *Mass Fatality and Casualty Incidents: A Field Guide.* Boca Raton, CRC Press (2011).

Johnson, B.T., & Riemen, J.A.J.M. Digital capture of fingerprints in a disaster victim identification setting: A review and case study. *Forensic Sciences Research* (2019), 4(4): 293–302.

Jonkman, S.N., & Kelman, I. An analysis of the causes and circumstances of flood disaster deaths. *Disasters* (2005), 29(1): 75–97.

Jutro, P. *How accurate are disaster movies?* 22 September 2012. https://peterjutro. com/how-accurate-are-disaster-movies/. Accessed 3 April 2022.

Leth, P.M. The use of CT scanning in forensic autopsy. *Forensic Science Medicine and Pathology* (2007), 3(1): 65–69.

Levinson, J. Interviews during various disasters. Unspecified for privacy reasons.

Maisel, D. (Vice President for Operations, United Hatzalah.) Interview with Levinson, in Jerusalem, 19 December 2021.

Makwana, N. Public health care system's preparedness to combat epidemics after natural disasters. *Journal of Family Medicine Primary Care* (2020), 9(10): 5107–5112.

Marshall, R.E., Milligan-Saville, J., Petrie, K., Bryant, R.A., Mitchell, P.B., & Harvey, S. Mental health screening amongst police officers: Factors associated with under-reporting of symptoms. *BMC Psychiatry* (2021), 21: 135.

Massey, K., & Sutton, J. Faith community's role in responding to disasters. *Southern Medical Journal* (2007), 100(9): 944–945.

Morrison, J., et al. Field-based detection of biological samples for forensic analysis: Established techniques, novel tools, and future innovations. *Forensic Science International* (2018), 285: 147–160.

National Institute of Justice. *A Guide for Explosion and Bombing Scene Investigation.* Washington, DC, National Institute of Justice (2000).

National Transportation Safety Board (NTSB). *Aircraft Accident Report Air Canada Flight 797 McDonnell Douglas Dc-9-32.* Washington, DC, NTSB (1983).

Nguyen, E., & Doyle, E. Dental post-mortem computed tomography for disaster victim identification: A literature review. *Journal of Forensic Radiology and Imaging* (2018), 13: 5–11.

O'Donnell, C., Iino, M., Mansharan, K., Leditscke, J., & Woodford, N. Contribution of postmortem multidetector CT scanning to identification of the deceased in a mass disaster: Experience gained from the 2009 Victorian bushfires. *Forensic Science International* (2011), 205(1–3): 15–28.

Ouyang, C., Zhou, K., Xu, Q., Yin, J., Peng, I.D., Wang, D., & Li, W. Dynamic analysis and numerical modeling of the 2015 catastrophic landslide of the construction waste landfill at Guangming, Shenzhen, China. *Landslides* (2017), 14: 705–718.

PAHO. *Management of Dead Bodies after Disasters: A Field Manual for First Responders* (2nd edition). Washington, DC, PAHO (2016).

Pescini, A. What we have learned from the Rigopiano tragedy. *Emergency Care Journal* (2019), 15(3).

Preparedex. *Internet.* www.preparedex.com/simulation-exercise-types-part-2/. Accessed 1 September 2021.

Riaud, X. Dr. Oscar Amoëdo Y Valdes (1863–1945), Founding father of forensic odontology. *Journal of Forensic Sciences & Criminal Investigation* (2017), 17(3): 5.

Rom, A., & Kelman, I. Search without rescue? Evaluating the international search and rescue response to earthquake disasters. *BMJ Global Health* (2020), 5.

Schwark, T., Heinrich, A., Preusse-Prange, A., & von Wurmb-Schwark, N. Reliable genetic identification of burnt human remains. *Forensic Science International Genetics* (2011), 5(5): 393–399

Shaw, G. A clinician's guide to digital X-ray systems. *Journal of the Royal Society of Medicine* (2001), 94(8): 391–395.

Sidler, M., Jackowski, C., Dirnhofer, R., Vock, P., & Thali, M. Use of multislice computed tomography in disaster victim identification—Advantages and limitations. *Forensic Science International* (2007), 169(2–3): 118–128

Silverthorne, J. *Morgue.* London, Stanley/Barker (2017).

Skinner, M., & Sterenberg, J. Turf wars: Authority and responsibility for the investigation of mass graves. *Forensic Science International* (2005), 151(2–3): 221–232.

SKYbrary. www.skybrary.aero/index.php/Smoke_Gases. Accessed 5 September 2021.

Smith, G.B., & Gordon, J.A. The admission of DNA evidence in State and federal courts, *Fordham Law Review* (1997), 65: 2465.

Speers, W.F. Rapid positive identification of fatal air disaster victims. *South African Medical Journal* (1977), 150.

Stadler, N. Terror, corpse symbolism, and taboo violation: The 'haredi disaster victim identification team in Israel' (Zaka). *Journal of the Royal Anthropological Institute* (2006), 12(4): 837–858.

Sweet, D. Interpol DVI best-practice standard: An overview. *Forensic Science International* (2010), 201(1–3): 18–21.

Tsaroom, S. Email correspondence with Levinson, 25 August 2021.

Tsaroom, S. *The Cloud Piller* (in Hebrew). Yehud-Monosson, Ofir Bikurim (2022).

Whittaker, J., McLennan, B., & Handmer, J. A review of informal volunteerism in emergencies and disasters: Definition, opportunities and challenges. *International Journal of Disaster Risk Reduction* (2010), 13(5): 358–368.

Wien, M., & Sabaté, J. Food selection criteria for disaster response planning in urban societies. *Nutrition Journal* (2015), 14: 47.

Wiersema, J.M., & Woody, A. The forensic anthropologist in the mass fatality context. *Academic Forensic Pathology* (2016), 6(3): 455–462.

Williams, J.A., & Weedn, V.W. (eds.). *Disaster Victim Identification in the 21st Century: A US Perspective.* Hoboken, New Jersey, Wiley (2022).

Zadok, A. Email correspondence with Levinson, 1 March 2022.

Zheng, J., Liu, N.G., & Chen, Y.J. The application of computed tomography (CT) in postmortem examination. *Fa Yi Xue Za Zhi* (2009), 25(4): 286–289.

Index

Note: Page numbers in *italics* indicate a figure on the corresponding page.

Printed in the United States
by Baker & Taylor Publisher Services